CLINICAL EMBRYOLOGY

VIDEO-INTEGRATED LEARNING RESOURCE FOR UNDERGRADUATE MEDICAL STUDENTS

DR. SHRIKANT AKOLEKAR

Made with ♥ on the Notion Press Platform
www.notionpress.com

Contents

Contents

Preface

This book comes from a series of Embryology lectures delivered to medical students in the Caribbean, especially those studying for the USMLE and NBME exams. Its scope, however, goes far beyond these settings and remains just as useful for professional exams in many other countries.

The digital revolution has profoundly reshaped the methods of teaching and learning. In response, these lectures have been adapted to a digital format while preserving the clarity of the textual narration for easier comprehension. The content is organized hierarchically, mirroring the natural progression of embryonic development from pre-fertilization events through the embryonic and fetal periods to maturity.

The book comprises 24 chapters, each structured with defined learning outcomes, a concise summary, and self-assessment questions to reinforce understanding. The material has been drawn from standard textbooks and carefully curated for accuracy, though occasional errors of omission or commission cannot be entirely excluded. Some of the Illustrations used in this manuscript have been generated using AI tools for educational purposes.

This concise resource is designed to bridge foundational principles with contemporary clinical relevance, offering medical students a streamlined yet comprehensive guide. The endeavor reflects a commitment to the free and accessible sharing of knowledge, rather than profit. The nominal price attached to the book serves only to cover digital maintenance costs.

I remain deeply grateful to my students and colleagues, whose questions, curiosity, and engagement have continually shaped the intellectual journey embodied in these pages.

Dr. Shrikant Akolekar
May 2026

Acknowledgements

Motto
"Tracing life's origins with clarity, from conception to Birth."

Acknowledgements

This E-Book would not have been possible without the support and collaboration of many individuals. I am thankful to my wife, Manik, whose unwavering support has been the foundation of my academic journey.

I extend heartfelt thanks to my students, past and present, whose curiosity, questions, and enthusiasm have shaped the structure and tone of this manuscript. Finally, I acknowledge the broader scientific community, researchers, clinicians, and educators whose collective efforts continue to expand our understanding of the nervous system. This book stands on the shoulders of their contributions.

I also extend my sincere thanks to Aishwarya and Jagadeeswar of Notion Press, whose dedicated support was instrumental in bringing this manuscript to life.

Note to Students

Embryology can sometimes feel abstract, but it is the foundation for understanding how the human body takes shape. This book has been prepared with you, the student, in mind. It is meant to simplify complex ideas, highlight the clinical connections, and guide you step by step through the fascinating journey of human development.

Each chapter begins with clear learning outcomes, ends with a summary to reinforce the essentials, and includes review questions to help you test your understanding. The goal is not only to prepare you for examinations but also to spark curiosity and confidence in applying embryological knowledge to clinical practice.

Think of this book as a companion on your path to becoming a thoughtful and skilled physician. Approach it with curiosity, revisit the diagrams and summaries often, and use the questions to challenge yourself.

This manuscript is a compilation of lectures delivered to students at various International Medical Universities in the Caribbean. The course content is clinically oriented and aligned with the requirements of USMLE/NBME-style examinations. Each chapter includes a hyperlink to the corresponding PowerPoint video presentation, which can be viewed on YouTube.

Corrigendum

Despite careful proofreading, a few errors remained in the published edition. The author regrets these inadvertent errors and any inconvenience they may have caused. Following the finalization of the manuscript, Chapters 5 and 10 were incorporated into the table of contents. As a result, the chapter numbering became misaligned with the corresponding video Learning sessions from Chapter 6 onward. The author regrets these oversights and appreciates the readers' understanding.

Part I Foundations of Human Embryology

CHAPTER I

Introduction to Clinical Embryology

Learning Objectives

By the end of this chapter, the student should be able to define embryology and explain its importance in medical practice; outline the major phases of human development from fertilization to birth; distinguish between the embryonic and fetal periods; explain the roles of gene regulation and epigenetic mechanisms in development; describe the principles of induction and intercellular signaling in organogenesis; and apply standard clinical terminology for gestational age and pregnancy periods.

Integrated Video Lecture

Video title: Introduction to Embryology
Hyperlink: https://youtu.be/AsVWyWmm4Os
Source: Private server

Scope and Clinical Relevance

Embryology is the scientific study of human development from a single fertilized cell to a fully formed individual. It forms a cornerstone of modern medicine because congenital anomalies represent a major global health burden. Each year, approximately 7.9 million infants are born with birth defects, making them one of the leading causes of infant morbidity and mortality worldwide. Advances in maternal care, prenatal screening, and neonatal management have reduced the incidence and severity of many anomalies, but a sound understanding of embryology remains essential for clinicians in obstetrics, pediatrics, surgery, radiology, and reproductive medicine.

Definition and Phases of Human Development

Embryology encompasses the molecular, cellular, and morphological processes that guide development from fertilization through the forty-week gestational period, culminating in birth.

Human development can be divided into two major phases.

The **pre-fertilization phase includes gametogenesis, the production and maturation of spermatozoa and oocytes, and** the preparation of the reproductive tracts for fertilization.

The **post-fertilization phase** is subdivided into the embryonic period, extending from fertilization to the end of the eighth week, during which the basic body plan and organ systems are established, and the fetal period, from the ninth week until birth, characterized by growth, tissue maturation, and functional refinement.

Cellular Processes in Development

Early embryonic development is driven by coordinated cellular events, including division, growth, migration, differentiation, rearrangement, and programmed cell death (apoptosis). These processes transform a single cell into a complex multicellular organism. The fetal period, in contrast, emphasizes growth and functional maturation, producing a viable fetus capable of independent survival.

Genetic Regulation

Nearly 19,500 protein-coding genes orchestrate human development within three billion nucleotides of DNA. Although all somatic cells contain the same genetic material, only selected genes are expressed at specific times and locations. Transcription factors regulate gene expression, either activating or repressing networks of genes. Among these, the **HOX genes** are highly conserved and critical for establishing the body plan, organ development, and limb formation. Mutations in HOX genes are linked to a wide range of congenital malformations.

Epigenetic Regulation

Gene expression is also controlled by epigenetic mechanisms, which alter function without changing DNA sequence. DNA methylation, histone modification, and chromatin remodeling ensure that specific cell types express appropriate proteins while silencing unrelated programs. For example, muscle cells express contractile proteins, while red blood cells express hemoglobin. These changes are stable yet reversible, allowing cells to adapt to developmental and environmental signals.

Induction and Intercellular Communication

Organogenesis depends on inductive interactions between tissues. An inducer sends signals that alter the fate of a responder, and this bidirectional crosstalk ensures coordinated differentiation, spatial organization, and functional integration.

Clinical Assessment of Gestational Age

Gestational age is conventionally calculated from the first day of the last menstrual period (LMP). A full-term pregnancy is defined as forty weeks, though ovulation and fertilization typically occur two weeks after the LMP, making the actual embryonic or fetal age approximately thirty-eight weeks.

The embryonic period spans weeks one to eight, while the fetal period extends from week nine to forty. This distinction is crucial for understanding teratogenic vulnerability, prenatal diagnosis, and clinical management.

Trimesters of Pregnancy

Pregnancy is divided into three trimesters. The first trimester (0–12 weeks) includes implantation, embryogenesis, and initiation of organ systems. The second trimester (13–28 weeks) is marked by organ development and fetal growth. The third trimester (29–40 weeks) involves rapid growth, fat deposition, and preparation for extrauterine life. Infants born before thirty-seven weeks are considered premature and may face complications such as respiratory distress.

Internal Genital Organs

The female internal genitalia include the ovaries, uterine tubes, uterus, and vagina. The male internal genitalia include the testes, epididymis, vas deferens, urethra, prostate, and seminal vesicles. These structures are essential for gametogenesis, fertilization, implantation, and reproduction.

Chapter Summary

Embryology is fundamental to understanding normal and abnormal human development. Human development occurs in embryonic and fetal phases, each with distinct characteristics. Gene regulation, HOX genes, and epigenetic mechanisms govern differentiation. Inductive signaling coordinates organ formation. Accurate assessment of gestational age is crucial for clinical practice.

Self-Assessment Questions

1. Define embryology and explain its clinical significance.
2. Differentiate between the embryonic and fetal periods.
3. Describe the role of HOX genes in development.
4. Explain how DNA methylation regulates gene expression.
5. How is gestational age calculated clinically?

CHAPTER II

Cytological Basis of Inheritance

Learning Objectives

By the end of this chapter, the student should be able to describe the structural and functional organization of human cells, explain the stages and regulation of the cell cycle, differentiate between mitosis and meiosis and their biological significance, describe the chromosomal basis of inheritance and its relation to Mendelian laws, define key genetic terms such as allele, locus, dominance, penetrance, and expressivity, and recognize the major modes of inheritance with their characteristic pedigree patterns.

Integrated Video Lecture

Video title: Cytological Basis of Inheritance
Hyperlink: https://youtu.be/UF2QoOjkMI0
Source: Private institutional server

Cellular Organization and Functional Principles

The human body is composed of trillions of cells organized into specialized tissues and integrated organ systems. Cells vary widely in size, shape, and internal organization, reflecting their diverse functional roles, yet they share a conserved structural plan. Each cell contains cytoplasm, which houses metabolic machinery and organelles, and one or more nuclei, which store genetic information in the form of DNA.

Somatic cells are governed by two fundamental imperatives: sustenance and propagation. Sustenance refers to metabolic processes that maintain cellular homeostasis and viability, while propagation refers to reproduction through division, ensuring continuity of genetic information.

The Cell Cycle

The life cycle of a eukaryotic cell consists of a series of orderly, regulated events that enable growth, DNA replication, and division. In most somatic cells, the cycle is divided into two major phases.

Interphase is the longest phase and includes the G1 phase, characterized by cellular growth and synthesis of RNA and proteins; the S phase, during which nuclear DNA is replicated; and the G2 phase, which prepares the cell for mitosis by synthesizing division machinery.

The **division phase** includes mitosis, the segregation of replicated chromosomes, and cytokinesis, the division of cytoplasm to form two genetically identical daughter cells. While many cells divide throughout life, certain cells, such as neurons, cardiac muscle cells, and skeletal muscle fibers, are largely non-dividing.

Types of Cell Division

Two distinct types of cell division occur in humans. **Mitosis**, or equational division, produces genetically identical daughter cells and is essential for growth, maintenance, and tissue repair. **Meiosis**, or reductional division, occurs in germ cells and results in haploid gametes, introducing genetic variability.

Chromosomal Basis of Inheritance

Inheritance is explained by the behavior of chromosomes during meiosis. Key events include pairing of homologous chromosomes, formation of chiasmata, and crossing over between chromatids. These processes result in genetic recombination, increasing variability among offspring. The movement and segregation of chromosomes during meiosis provide the physical basis for Mendel's laws of segregation and independent assortment.

Alleles and Gene Expression

Genes occupying corresponding positions on homologous chromosomes are known as alleles. Alleles may be identical (homozygous) or different (heterozygous). A heterozygous individual may be phenotypically normal, acting as a carrier, or affected, depending on the dominance relationships of the alleles involved.

Dominance, Penetrance, and Expressivity

A dominant trait is expressed in heterozygous individuals, while a recessive trait is expressed only when both alleles are recessive. **Expressivity** refers to the degree or intensity with which a trait manifests in an individual. **Penetrance** refers to the proportion of individuals with a specific genotype who exhibit the phenotype. Complete penetrance means the trait is always expressed, whereas incomplete penetrance means it is expressed in only some individuals.

Categories of Genetic Disorders

Genetic disorders are broadly classified into three groups. **Single-gene disorders** result from mutations in a single gene. **Chromosomal disorders** arise from numerical or structural abnormalities. **Multifactorial disorders** result from interactions between multiple genes and environmental factors.

Modes of Inheritance Single-gene disorders follow specific inheritance patterns.

Autosomal dominant inheritance is characterized by vertical transmission across generations, equal frequency in males and females, and absence of transmission by unaffected individuals. It often involves genes encoding structural proteins. Examples include Huntington disease, achondroplasia, neurofibromatosis, and familial hypercholesterolemia.

Autosomal recessive inheritance occurs when affected individuals inherit two mutant alleles. Parents are typically asymptomatic carriers, and the trait often appears among siblings rather than parents. It shows equal sex distribution, a recurrence risk of 25%, and increased frequency with consanguinity. Examples include sickle cell disease, cystic fibrosis, and phenylketonuria.

X-linked inheritance may be dominant or recessive. In **X-linked dominant inheritance**, females are more frequently affected, there is no father-to-son transmission, and all daughters of affected males are affected. Examples include vitamin D–resistant rickets, Rett syndrome, and fragile X syndrome.

In **X-linked recessive inheritance**, males are more commonly affected, carrier females transmit the disease, and inheritance often follows a pattern from affected grandfathers to carrier daughters to affected grandsons. Examples include Hemophilia A and B and Duchenne muscular dystrophy.

Mitochondrial inheritance involves mitochondrial DNA, which contains thirty-seven genes essential for oxidative phosphorylation. Mitochondria are inherited exclusively from the mother, so both sons and daughters may be affected, but only females transmit the condition. Clinical severity varies due to heteroplasmy. Examples include Leber hereditary optic neuropathy and Leigh syndrome.

Chapter Summary

Cells maintain life through metabolism and propagation. The cell cycle regulates growth, DNA replication, and division. Meiosis provides the chromosomal basis for inheritance and genetic variation. Patterns of inheritance explain the transmission of genetic disorders. Understanding inheritance patterns is fundamental to diagnosis and genetic counseling.

Self-Assessment Questions

1. Differentiate mitosis from meiosis.
2. Explain the chromosomal basis of Mendel's laws.
3. Define penetrance and expressivity.
4. List the hallmarks of autosomal recessive inheritance.
5. Why is mitochondrial inheritance exclusively maternal?

CHAPTER III

Gametogenesis

Learning Objectives

By the end of this chapter, the student should be able to define gametogenesis and distinguish between spermatogenesis and oogenesis, describe the stages and regulation of oocyte development from fetal life to fertilization, explain the endocrine regulation of follicular development and ovulation, describe the stages of spermatogenesis and spermiogenesis, compare the structural and functional specializations of male and female gametes, and apply foundational knowledge of meiosis and gamete maturation to clinical scenarios.

Integrated Video Lecture
Video title: Gametogenesis
Hyperlink: https://youtu.be/h2r_4o_EvO4
Source: Private institutional server

Overview of Gametogenesis

Gametogenesis is the process by which male and female germ cells undergo meiotic division and cytodifferentiation to form haploid gametes—spermatozoa in males and oocytes in females. Primordial germ cells are diploid, each containing 23 pairs of chromosomes. Through two meiotic divisions, the chromosome number is reduced to 23, preparing gametes for fertilization. Although both gametes arise through meiosis, oogenesis and spermatogenesis follow distinct temporal patterns and differentiation pathways.

Part I: Oogenesis

Oogenesis begins during fetal life. By the twelfth week of gestation, oogonia undergo rapid mitotic proliferation, forming up to seven million primary oocytes. Each primary oocyte enters meiosis I and arrests at the diplotene stage of prophase I, a state that persists for years. At birth, approximately three million primary oocytes remain; by puberty, only about 400,000 survive due to atresia. Over the reproductive lifespan, 400–500 oocytes are ovulated, while the remainder undergo hormonally regulated apoptosis.

At puberty, cyclical hormonal signals allow a cohort of oocytes to resume meiosis. At ovulation, the primary oocyte completes meiosis I, forming a secondary oocyte and the first polar body. The secondary oocyte immediately enters meiosis II but arrests at metaphase II until fertilization. Upon fertilization, meiosis II is completed, the second polar body is extruded, and the female pronucleus is formed. Each primary oocyte ultimately yields one mature ovum and two or three polar bodies, reflecting the cytoplasmic conservation strategy of oogenesis.

Oogenesis is regulated by the hypothalamic–pituitary–ovarian axis. Pulsatile release of GnRH from the hypothalamus stimulates FSH and LH secretion from the anterior pituitary. FSH promotes follicular growth and estrogen synthesis via granulosa cells, while LH acts on theca cells and later luteinized granulosa cells to stimulate progesterone synthesis. Rising FSH recruits follicles but falling levels lead to atresia of all but one dominant follicle. The LH surge triggers ovulation, completing the cycle of follicular recruitment and dominance.

Part II: Spermatogenesis

Spermatogenesis begins at puberty and continues throughout life, requiring approximately 64 days for completion. It is divided into three phases: spermatocytogenesis, meiosis, and spermiogenesis.

Stem cell populations include type A dark spermatogonia, which serve as dormant reserves; type A pale spermatogonia, which renew through mitosis; and type B spermatogonia, which differentiate into primary spermatocytes. Primary spermatocytes undergo meiosis I to form secondary spermatocytes, which then complete meiosis II to produce spermatids.

Spermiogenesis transforms spermatids into mature spermatozoa through nuclear condensation, loss of excess cytoplasm, formation of the acrosome, development of the flagellum, and mitochondrial concentration in the midpiece.

Mature spermatozoa enter the epididymis, where they acquire motility.

Sertoli cells provide structural and metabolic support, form the blood–testis barrier, facilitate germ cell movement, and secrete androgen-binding protein and inhibin. Leydig cells, located in the interstitial tissue, produce testosterone, essential for spermatogenesis and male phenotype development.

Normal sperm counts range from 60–200 million/ml. Oligospermia refers to counts of 10–20 million/mL, while severe oligospermia is defined as fewer than 5 million/ml. Each primary spermatocyte produces four mature spermatozoa, in contrast to the single ovum produced by oogenesis.

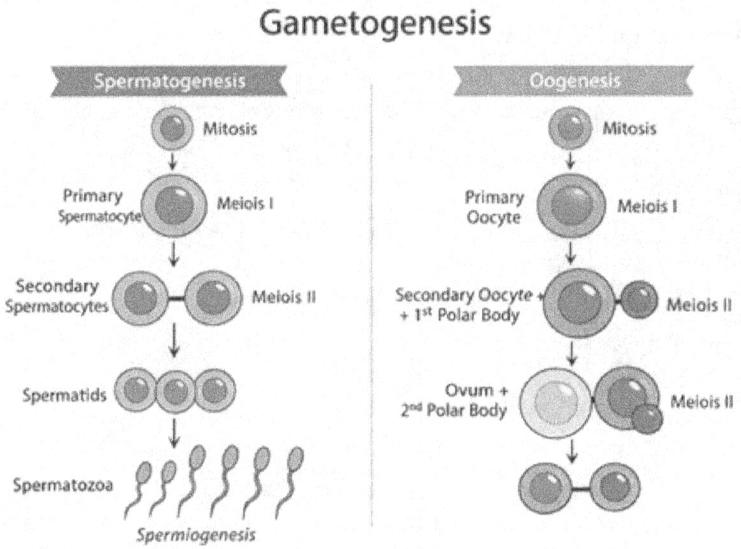

Part III: Functional Comparison of Gametes

Sperm are specialized for motility, contain enzymes for zona pellucida penetration, and exhibit receptor-mediated recognition of the oocyte. They have minimal cytoplasm. Oocytes, in contrast, contain abundant cytoplasmic determinants, attract sperm via chemoattraction, deploy blocks to polyspermy, and provide the metabolic substrates required for early embryonic development. These complementary adaptations ensure efficient fertilization and initiation of embryogenesis.

Chapter Summary

Gametogenesis involves meiotic reduction and cytodifferentiation to produce haploid gametes. Oogenesis begins in fetal life and is hormonally regulated throughout the reproductive lifespan. Spermatogenesis begins at puberty and continues throughout life, producing large numbers of sperm. The hypothalamic–pituitary–ovarian axis coordinates oocyte maturation and ovulation. Sperm and oocytes exhibit distinct structural and functional adaptations essential for fertilization.

Self-Assessment Questions

1. Describe the major differences between oogenesis and spermatogenesis.
2. At what stage is the secondary oocyte arrested, and how is meiosis II completed?
3. Explain the role of FSH and LH in follicular development.
4. Outline the stages of spermiogenesis.
5. What features distinguish the mature spermatozoon from the mature ovum?

MCQ 1

A 32-year-old woman has an increased risk of conceiving a child with trisomy 21. Which of the following is the most likely underlying mechanism?

A. Failure of spermiogenesis
B. Nondisjunction during meiosis I
C. Failure of fertilization
D. Mitotic arrest of the zygote
E. Abnormal implantatio

Correct Answer: B

Explanation:
Advanced maternal age is associated with **meiotic nondisjunction**, most commonly during **meiosis I**, leading to aneuploidy such as trisomy 21.

MCQ 2

A defect in spermatogenesis results in the formation of immature spermatozoa that fail to acquire motility. Which process is most likely impaired?

A. Spermiation
B. Spermatocytogenesis
C. Spermiogenesis
D. Meiosis II
E. Capacitation

Answer: C

Explanation:
Spermiogenesis is the transformation of spermatids into mature spermatozoa, including the development of motility and acrosome formation.

CHAPTER IV

Ovulation to Implantation

First Week of Development

Learning Objectives

By the end of this chapter, the student should be able to describe the phases of the menstrual cycle and their endocrine regulation, explain the processes of ovulation, oocyte transport, and sperm capacitation, describe the sequential phases of fertilization and their molecular mechanisms, outline cleavage, morula formation, blastocyst formation, and hatching, explain the process and timing of implantation and trophoblast differentiation, describe early placental formation, decidual changes, and chorionic villi development, and recognize early developmental anomalies such as ectopic pregnancy, twin types, and hydatidiform mole.

Integrated Video Lectures
Part 1: Ovulation to Fertilization
Part 2: Cleavage to Implantation and Early Placentation
Hyperlink: https://youtu.be/Sm8ZnKmMnjU

The Menstrual Cycle

Menarche typically occurs between ages twelve and fourteen, marking the onset of reproductive capacity. The reproductive period extends from adolescence to approximately forty-five years and is characterized by cyclic events recurring every twenty-five to thirty-five days, with an average of twenty-eight days. These changes constitute the menstrual cycle, a coordinated sequence that prepares the endometrium for potential implantation.

The cycle consists of three phases. The **follicular phase** is driven by FSH, leading to follicular growth, estrogen secretion, and endometrial proliferation. **Ovulation** occurs around day fourteen, triggered by the mid-cycle LH surge, resulting in the release of a metaphase II secondary oocyte. The **luteal phase** follows, during which the corpus luteum secretes progesterone, rendering the endometrium secretory and receptive to implantation. If fertilization does not occur, steroid hormone levels fall, leading to menstruation.

Endocrine Regulation of Ovulation

The menstrual cycle is regulated by the hypothalamic–pituitary–ovarian axis. Pulsatile release of GnRH from the hypothalamus stimulates FSH and LH secretion from the anterior pituitary. FSH acts on granulosa cells to promote estrogen production, while LH acts on theca cells to provide androgen substrates for estrogen synthesis. The LH surge induces ovulation and luteinization. After follicle rupture, the oocyte is captured by the fimbriae of the uterine tube and enters the ampulla, the usual site of fertilization.

Sperm Capacitation and Transport

Ejaculation occurs in two phases: emission, the delivery of semen to the prostatic urethra, and expulsion, coordinated by somatic and autonomic mechanisms. Post-ejaculation events include semen coagulation, liquefaction within fifteen to twenty minutes, neutralization of vaginal acidity by alkaline seminal fluid, and sperm migration through cervical mucus. Capacitation, a seven-hour process involving removal of the glycoprotein coat and acrosomal proteins, is essential for zona pellucida penetration. Only a small fraction of sperm reach the ampulla, where fertilization occurs.

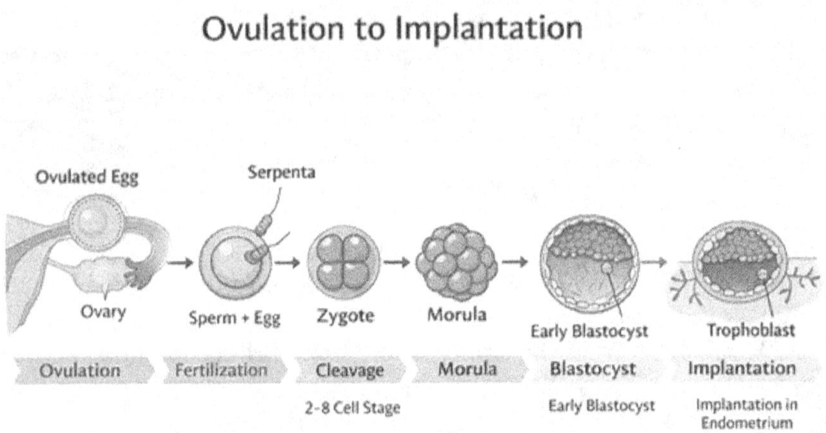

Development of the Embryo (Fertilization to Blastocyst): *Sequential stages from fertilization to implantation, showing zygote cleavage, morula formation, and blastocyst differentiation into trophoblast and inner cell mass.*
This diagram illustrates the earliest events of human development. Following fertilization, the zygote undergoes rapid mitotic divisions, forming the morula, which then develops into the blastocyst. The outer trophoblast contributes to the placenta, while the inner cell mass forms the embryo proper. Understanding these transitions clarifies how cellular specialization begins even before implantation, establishing the foundation for embryonic and extra-embryonic structures.

Fertilization

Fertilization proceeds through three phases. First, sperm penetrate the corona radiata, aided by flagellar activity and hyaluronidase. Second, sperm bind to ZP3 receptors on the zona pellucida, triggering the acrosomal reaction and enzymatic digestion that allows penetration. Third, fusion of the oolemma and sperm initiates the cortical reaction, preventing polyspermy. The male pronucleus forms, while the secondary oocyte completes meiosis II to form the female pronucleus and a second polar body. Fusion of the pronuclei restores the diploid chromosome number, producing a zygote and initiating embryogenesis.

Cleavage and Morula Formation

Cleavage divisions begin immediately after fertilization. On day one, the zygote reaches the two-cell stage; by day two, the four-cell stage; and by day three, the eight-cell stage. These blastomeres are totipotent. At the eight- to sixteen-cell stage, compaction occurs, with increased adhesion, tight junction formation, and polarity between outer and inner cell masses. By day four, the morula forms, a compact ball of twelve to thirty-two cells. The outer cell mass becomes the trophoblast, while the inner cell mass becomes the embryoblast. E-cadherin plays a critical role in compaction.

Blastocyst Formation and Hatching

By days four to five, the morula enters the uterine cavity, where fluid accumulation creates the blastocyst cavity. The embryoblast forms the future embryo, while the trophoblast develops into the placenta. Hatching occurs between days five and six, as the blastocyst escapes the zona pellucida through enzymatic digestion, uterine contractions, and hydrostatic pressure. Hatching is essential for implantation.

Implantation

Implantation begins on days six to seven, when the blastocyst attaches to the posterior superior uterine wall. The trophoblast differentiates into two layers: the cytotrophoblast, a mitotically active inner layer, and the syncytiotrophoblast, an invasive multinucleated outer layer. The syncytiotrophoblast invades the endometrial stroma, erodes maternal vessels and glands, and begins secreting hCG. This hormone maintains corpus luteum progesterone secretion and forms the basis of pregnancy tests, detectable in serum by day nine and in urine by day twelve to fourteen.

Early Placentation and Decidual Reaction

Between days eight and ten, lacunae form within the syncytiotrophoblast and fill with maternal blood, initiating primitive uteroplacental circulation. By days thirteen to fourteen, cytotrophoblast cells proliferate into the syncytiotrophoblast, forming primary chorionic villi that later vascularize to establish the definitive placenta. Decidualization of endometrial stromal cells produces three regions: the decidua basalis, the maternal component of the placenta; the decidua capsularis, covering the implanted embryo; and the decidua parietalis, comprising the remaining endometrium.

Bilaminar Germ Disc and Cavities

Within the embryoblast, the amniotic cavity forms. The embryoblast differentiates into epiblast and hypoblast, creating the bilaminar embryonic disc. The yolk sac develops in two stages: the primary yolk sac, lined by the exocoelomic membrane, and the definitive yolk sac, formed by migrating hypoblast cells. Extraembryonic mesoderm fills the space between trophoblast and yolk/amniotic sacs, and cavities merge to form the extraembryonic coelom, or chorionic cavity. The connecting stalk emerges as the primordium of the umbilical cord. At this stage, the amnion, chorion, and yolk sac are established.

Early Developmental Anomalies

Ectopic pregnancy occurs when implantation takes place outside the uterine cavity, most commonly in the fallopian tube. Tubal rupture risk increases with gestation, and rare cases involve abdominal implantation. Twins may be monozygotic, arising from a single zygote and genetically identical, or dizygotic, resulting from fertilization of two oocytes by two sperm. Conjoined twins result from incomplete division of the embryonic disc, with types including craniopagus, Thoracopagus, Omphalopagus, and Ischiopagus. A hydatidiform mole arises from abnormal fertilization, often polyspermy, leading to excessive trophoblastic proliferation and elevated maternal hCG. Complete and partial forms exist, with clinical importance due to the risk of gestational trophoblastic disease.

Chapter Summary

Week one spans from ovulation to implantation. Fertilization occurs in the ampulla and involves sequential steps of penetration and fusion. Cleavage and morula formation precede blastocyst formation and hatching. Implantation begins on days six to seven and requires trophoblast differentiation. hCG secretion maintains pregnancy and enables early detection. Early anomalies include ectopic pregnancy, twins, and molar pregnancy.

Self-Assessment Questions

1. Describe the phases of the menstrual cycle and their hormonal regulation.
2. Explain the three phases of fertilization.
3. What are the roles of the cytotrophoblast and syncytiotrophoblast in implantation?
4. Outline the sequence from zygote to morula to blastocyst.
5. What are the differences between complete and partial hydatidiform moles?

MCQs

1.The trophoblast of the blastocyst primarily contributes to:

A. Embryo proper
B. Placenta
C. Amnion
D. Yolk sac

Answer: B

2. The morula stage is characterized by:

A. Formation of three germ layers
B. A solid ball of blastomeres
C. Differentiation into trophoblast and inner cell mass
D. Implantation into the uterine wall

Answer: B

3. A sperm is unable to penetrate the zona pellucida despite normal motility. Which structure is most likely defective?

A. Flagellum

B. Acrosome
C. Nucleus
D. Mitochondria
E. Centriole

Answer: B

Explanation:
The **acrosome** contains enzymes required for penetration of the zona pellucida.

4. A fertilized ovum fails to prevent the entry of additional sperm. Which mechanism has failed?

A. Capacitation
B. Cortical reaction
C. Cleavage
D. Gastrulation
E. Implantation

Answer: B

Explanation:
The **cortical reaction** modifies the zona pellucida to prevent polyspermy.

5. A pregnancy test detects elevated hCG levels. Which cells are responsible for its production?

A. Cytotrophoblast
B. Syncytiotrophoblast
C. Epiblast
D. Hypoblast
E. Decidua basalis

Answer: B

6. An ectopic pregnancy is most commonly located in which region?

A. Cervix
B. Ovary
C. Ampulla of the uterine tube
D. Isthmus
E. Peritoneal cavity

Answer: C

CHAPTER V

Development of the Fetal Membranes (Week) (Amnion, Chorion, Yolk Sac, and Allantois)

Learning Objectives

By the end of this chapter, the student should be able to describe the origin and development of the amnion, chorion, yolk sac, and allantois, explain their roles in supporting embryonic and fetal development, outline the structural and functional changes of each membrane across gestation, correlate their contributions to placental and umbilical cord formation, and recognize clinical anomalies associated with fetal membrane development.

Integrated Video Lecture
Video title: Development of the Fetal Membranes
Hyperlink: https://youtu.be/WK7qof1jeRI
Source: Private institutional server

Introduction

Fetal membranes are extraembryonic structures that develop alongside the embryo and play essential roles in protection, nutrition, waste removal, and gas exchange. They include the amnion, chorion, yolk sac, and allantois. Together, these membranes form the environment in which the embryo grows and contribute to the placenta and umbilical cord.

The Amnion

The amnion arises from the epiblast and extraembryonic somatic mesoderm. By the second week, the amniotic cavity forms within the embryoblast, lined by amnioblasts. The amniotic sac expands rapidly, eventually surrounding the embryo and filling with amniotic fluid.

Functions of the Amnion and Amniotic Fluid

- Cushions the embryo against mechanical injury
- Permits symmetrical growth and free movement
- Prevents adhesions between the embryo and surrounding tissues
- Maintains a stable temperature
- Facilitates lung development through fetal breathing movements

Clinical note: Oligohydramnios (too little fluid) and polyhydramnios (too much fluid) are associated with congenital anomalies such as renal agenesis and gastrointestinal obstruction, respectively.

The Chorion

The chorion develops from trophoblast and extraembryonic mesoderm. Initially, villi cover the entire chorionic sac. By week eight, villi near the decidua basalis proliferate to form the chorion frondosum, while those near the decidua capsularis degenerate, forming the chorion laeve. The chorion contributes to the fetal portion of the placenta and plays a central role in establishing uteroplacental circulation. Its villous structures mediate maternal–fetal exchange.

The Yolk Sac

The yolk sac is the first extraembryonic structure to appear, forming during the second week. The primary yolk sac is lined by the exocoelomic membrane, later replaced by the definitive yolk sac formed by migrating hypoblast cells.

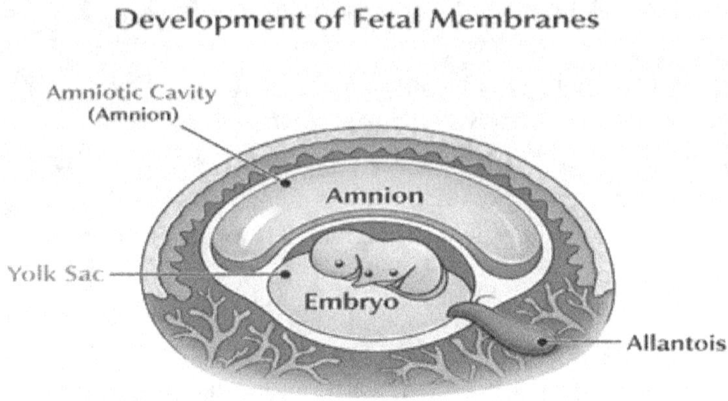

Development of Fetal Membranes *showing the formation and spatial relationships of the amnion, chorion, yolk sac, and allantois around the embryo. The chorionic cavity disappears shortly as the amniotic cavity expands to fill the entire space. The amnion and chorion fuse to form a single amniochorionic cavity.*

Functions of the Yolk Sac

- Early hematopoiesis (weeks 3–6)
- Origin of primordial germ cells
- Contribution to the formation of the midgut via incorporation during folding
- Nutrient transfer in early development

Clinical note: Persistent vitelline duct remnants may lead to Meckel's diverticulum, a common congenital anomaly of the small intestine.

The Allantois

The allantois appears around day sixteen as a diverticulum of the yolk sac extending into the connecting stalk. Although vestigial in humans, it plays important roles in early development.

Functions of the Allantois

- Contributes to the formation of the umbilical vessels
- Participates in early blood formation
- Forms the urachus, which later becomes the median umbilical ligament

Clinical note: Patent urachus may result in urine leakage from the umbilicus.

Integration into Placenta and Umbilical Cord

The fetal membranes integrate to form the placenta and umbilical cord. The chorion frondosum becomes the fetal placenta, the amnion fuses with the chorion to form the amnio chorionic membrane, and the yolk sac and allantois contribute to the umbilical vessels and cord structure. The umbilical cord ultimately contains two arteries, one vein, Wharton's jelly, and vestigial remnants of the yolk sac and allantois.

Chapter Summary

The fetal membranes, amnion, chorion, yolk sac, and allantois develop early in gestation and provide essential support for embryonic and fetal life. The amnion protects the embryo, the chorion forms the fetal placenta, the yolk sac supports early hematopoiesis and germ cell origin, and the allantois contributes to umbilical vessel formation. Their integration ensures proper placental function and umbilical cord development. Abnormalities such as oligohydramnios, Meckel's diverticulum, and patent urachus highlight their clinical relevance.

Self-Assessment Questions

1. What are the origins and functions of the amnion?
2. How does the chorion contribute to placental development?
3. What are the roles of the yolk sac in early embryogenesis?
4. Describe the developmental fate of the allantois.

5. How do the fetal membranes integrate into the placenta and umbilical cord?
6. What clinical anomalies are associated with yolk sac and allantois remnants?

MCQs

1. The yolk sac plays a critical role in:

A. Placental exchange
B. Early hematopoiesis
C. Neural crest migration
D. Amniotic fluid production

Answer: B

2. The amnion is derived from:

A. Endoderm
B. Mesoderm
C. Ectoderm
D. Trophoblast

Answer: C

3. The epiblast gives rise to which of the following structures?

A. Amnion
B. Yolk sac lining
C. Cytotrophoblast
D. Chorion
E. Decidua

Answer: A

CHAPTER VI

Gastrulation (Week 3)

Learning Objectives

By the end of this chapter, the student should be able to define gastrulation and describe its role in establishing the body plan, identify the structures formed during gastrulation including the primitive streak, node, and pit, describe the formation and derivatives of the three primary germ layers, explain the formation, function, and fate of the notochord, outline the differentiation of the intraembryonic mesoderm into paraxial, intermediate, and lateral plate regions, describe somite formation and explain the derivatives of sclerotome, myotome, and dermatome, explain cavitation of the lateral plate mesoderm and formation of the intraembryonic coelom, and recognize congenital anomalies associated with abnormalities of gastrulation.

Integrated Video Lecture
Video title: Gastrulation
Hyperlink: https://youtu.be/JEgPmUwHmHw
Source: Private institutional server

Overview of Gastrulation

Gastrulation marks the beginning of body plan establishment in human development. It transforms the bilaminar germ disc, composed of epiblast and hypoblast, into a trilaminar disc consisting of ectoderm, mesoderm, and endoderm. These three germ layers give rise to all tissues and organ systems. Gastrulation begins in the third week of development and involves coordinated changes in cell shape, proliferation, epithelial-to-mesenchymal transition, and directed migration.

Formation of the Primitive Streak

The earliest morphological sign of gastrulation is the primitive streak, a midline thickened band of proliferating epiblast cells in the caudal region of the embryonic disc. As the streak elongates cranially, the primitive node forms at its anterior end, a primitive groove develops along its length, and a primitive pit appears within the node. These structures regulate cell migration and patterning during germ layer formation.

Germ Layer Formation

Epiblast cells migrate toward the primitive streak, invaginate, and move between the epiblast and hypoblast. The first cells to invaginate displace the hypoblast and form the definitive endoderm. Subsequent waves spread laterally and cranially to form the intraembryonic mesoderm, which is absent at the prechordal plate and cloacal membrane. Epiblast cells that remain on the dorsal surface become ectoderm. By the end of the third week, the trilaminar germ disc is established.

Formation and Significance of the Notochord

Cells migrating cranially from the primitive node form the notochord, a midline rod-like structure extending toward the prechordal plate. The notochord defines the embryonic axis, provides signals for neural induction, influences paraxial mesoderm differentiation, and establishes the template for the vertebral column. Although most of the notochord regresses as vertebral bodies develop, a remnant persists as the nucleus pulposus of the intervertebral disc.

Differentiation of the Intraembryonic Mesoderm

During the third week, the intraembryonic mesoderm differentiates into three regions.

The **paraxial mesoderm**, located adjacent to the notochord, gives rise to somites. Somites form in a craniocaudal sequence beginning around day twenty-one, at a rate of three pairs per day, ultimately producing thirty-four pairs. Somites differentiate into sclerotome, which forms vertebrae and ribs; myotome, which forms skeletal musculature; and dermatome, which forms the dermis of the skin.

The **intermediate mesoderm** develops into the urogenital system, including kidneys, ureters, gonads, and reproductive ducts.

The **lateral plate mesoderm** undergoes cavitation to form the intraembryonic coelom. It divides into somatic mesoderm, which contributes to the body wall, limbs, parietal serous membranes, and amnion, and splanchnic mesoderm, which forms the heart, blood vessels, smooth muscle, and connective tissue of the gut and respiratory system, and visceral serous membranes. The coelom ultimately becomes the pericardial, pleural, and peritoneal cavities.

Somitogenesis

Somites form in a precise sequence, establishing the early segmental organization of the embryo. Somitomeres one to seven contribute to skeletal and muscular components of the head and neck, while the remaining Somitomeres form thirty-four somite pairs. Somite derivatives include sclerotome, which forms vertebrae, ribs, and part of the occipital bone; myotome, which divides into epimere (deep back muscles) and hypomere (trunk and limb muscles); and dermatome, which forms the dermis of the dorsal body wall.

Formation of the Intraembryonic Coelom

Cavitation within the lateral plate mesoderm produces intercellular spaces that coalesce into the intraembryonic coelom. This separates somatic and splanchnic mesoderm, partitions the embryonic body, and gives rise to all major cavities. Somatic mesoderm lines the amnion and forms the body wall, limbs, and parietal layers of serous membranes. Splanchnic mesoderm forms connective tissue and smooth muscle of the gut and respiratory organs, visceral serous membranes, blood vessels, and the heart.

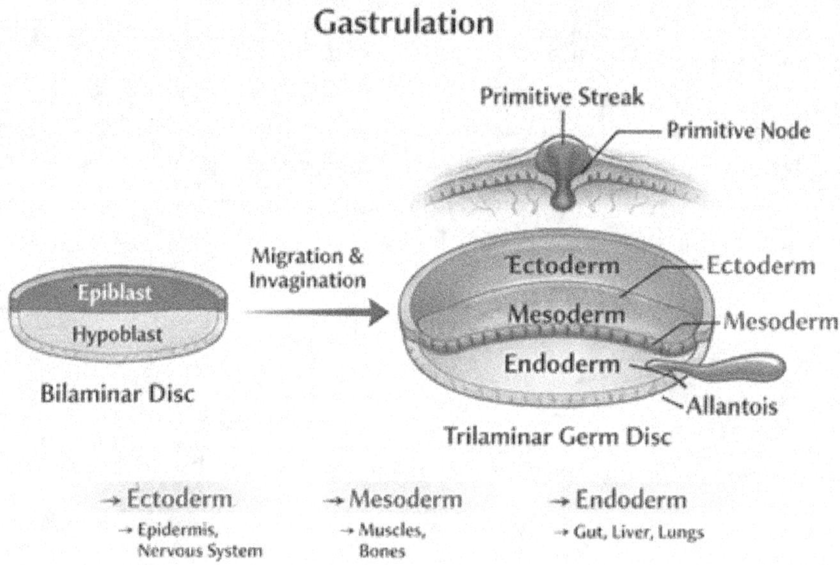

Regression of the Primitive Streak and Clinical Correlation

By the fourth week, the primitive streak regresses and disappears. Persistence of streak remnants can lead to sacrococcygeal teratoma, the most common tumor in newborns. These tumors contain pluripotent cells capable of differentiating into multiple tissue types. They are typically located at the base of the spine, often benign, but may require surgical removal.

Chapter Summary

Gastrulation transforms the bilaminar disc into a trilaminar embryo. The primitive streak, node, and pit regulate cell migration and patterning. Ectoderm, mesoderm, and endoderm give rise to all tissues of the embryo. Notochord formation defines the embryonic axis and induces neural differentiation. Mesoderm differentiates into paraxial, intermediate, and lateral plate regions. Somitogenesis establishes early metamerism and gives rise to musculoskeletal components. Cavitation of the lateral plate mesoderm forms the intraembryonic coelom. Failure of primitive streak regression may lead to sacrococcygeal teratoma.

Self-Assessment Questions

1. What structures develop from the three primary germ layers?
2. Describe the stages of primitive streak formation.
3. Explain the role of the notochord in early development.
4. List the derivatives of paraxial, intermediate, and lateral plate mesoderm.
5. How is the intraembryonic coelom formed?

MCQs

1. A defect in the formation of the primitive streak can lead to:

A. Holoprosencephaly
B. Sirenomelia
C. Cleft palate
D. Spina bifida
E. Tetralogy of Fallot

Answer: B

2. Which germ layer gives rise to skeletal muscle?

A. Ectoderm
B. Mesoderm
C. Endoderm
D. Neural crest
E. Placodal cells

Answer: B

CHAPTER VII

Neurulation (Week 3)

Learning Objectives

By the end of this chapter, the student should be able to define neurulation and distinguish between primary and secondary neurulation, describe the formation, folding, and closure of the neural tube, explain the formation, migration, and derivatives of neural crest cells, identify the timing of cranial and caudal neuropore closure and associated anomalies, outline the development of the brain vesicles and early CNS flexures, describe the embryologic origins of the meninges and ventricular system, and recognize congenital anomalies arising from defective neurulation.

Integrated Video Lecture
Video title: Neurulation
Hyperlink: https://youtu.be/cyM9H_j1ou8
Source: Private institutional server

Overview of Neurulation

Neurulation is the embryonic process that establishes the central nervous system. Beginning in the third week, shortly after gastrulation, the ectoderm thickens to form the neural plate. This marks the initiation of primary neurulation, in which the neural plate folds and fuses to form the neural tube.

Formation of the Neural Plate

Around day eighteen, the surface ectoderm proliferates and thickens in the midline, forming the neural plate. This structure extends cranially and is widest at the future head region, where the brain will develop.

Primary Neurulation: Folding and Fusion

Neural tube formation proceeds through sequential morphological changes.

By days eighteen to nineteen, the neural plate invaginates to form the neural groove, with lateral edges elevating as neural folds. By day twenty, the folds converge toward the midline, and fusion begins in the cervical region, progressing cranially and caudally. Fusion converts the groove into a closed neural tube, which separates from the overlying ectoderm. The surface ectoderm then reestablishes continuity, forming the future epidermis.

Neuropores and Timing of Closure

At the time of fusion, the cranial and caudal ends remain open as neuropores. The cranial neuropore closes between days twenty-three and twenty-six; failure results in anencephaly, a lethal condition characterized by the absence of the cranial vault and exposed neural tissue. The caudal neuropore closes between days twenty-six and twenty-nine; failure results in spina bifida, ranging from occult forms to open defects such as meningocele and meningomyelocele. Rarely, complete failure of closure produces craniorachischisis, a lethal anomaly involving both brain and spinal cord.

Neural Crest Cells

During neural fold fusion, crest cells undergo epithelial-to-mesenchymal transition and form the neural crest, a multipotent migratory population. Neural crest derivatives include dorsal root and cranial nerve sensory ganglia, autonomic ganglia, Schwann cells, and enteric ganglia. They also contribute to craniofacial bones and cartilage, odontoblasts, chromaffin cells of the adrenal medulla, thyroid parafollicular cells, melanocytes, pia and arachnoid mater, and cells involved in outflow tract septation of the heart.

Clinical correlations include Hirschsprung disease, caused by failure of neural crest migration to the distal colon, and Waardenburg syndrome, characterized by pigmentary abnormalities, sensorineural hearing loss, and a white forelock due to defective crest migration and differentiation.

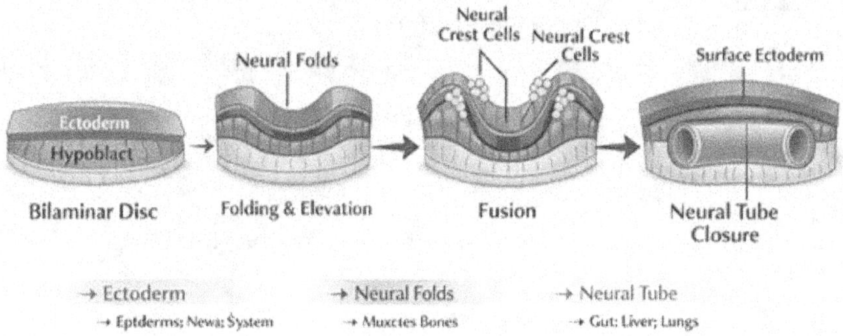

***Neurulation**, illustrating the sequential transformation from the neural plate to the closed neural tube. It shows the four key stages: **neural plate formation, elevation of neural folds, fusion at the midline, and closure of the neural tube**, with neural crest cells highlighted at the margins.*

Differentiation of the Neural Tube

After closure, the cranial two-thirds of the neural tube form the brain, while the caudal one-third forms the spinal cord. The central canal persists as the ventricular system.

Development of Brain Vesicles

By the end of the fourth week, three primary brain vesicles are evident: the prosencephalon (forebrain), mesencephalon (midbrain), and rhombencephalon (hindbrain). Flexures develop, including the cephalic flexure between midbrain and forebrain, and the cervical flexure between hindbrain and spinal cord.

By week five, the vesicles differentiate further. The prosencephalon forms the telencephalon, giving rise to cerebral hemispheres, basal ganglia, olfactory system, and lateral ventricles, and the diencephalon, which forms the thalamus, hypothalamus, epithalamus, subthalamus, and the third ventricle. The mesencephalon remains undivided, forming the midbrain and cerebral aqueduct. The rhombencephalon divides into metencephalon (pons) and myelencephalon (medulla), with the rhombic lip forming the cerebellum. The cavity becomes the fourth ventricle.

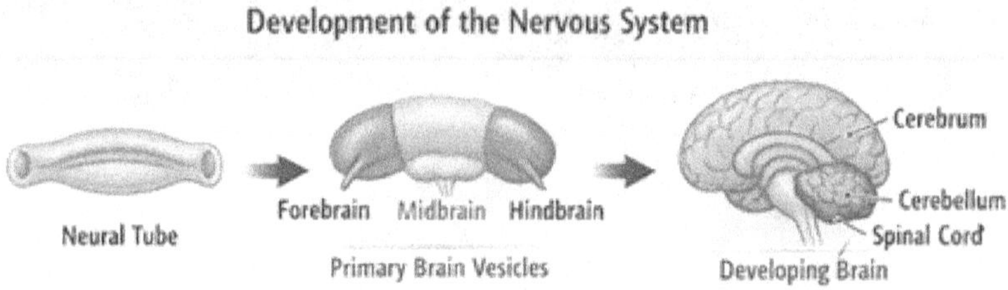

Development of the Nervous System*, illustrating the transformation of the* ***neural tube*** *into the* ***brain and spinal cord****, and the emergence of the* ***peripheral nervous system***

Meningeal Development

The meninges arise from two sources. Neural crest cells form the pia and arachnoid mater, while mesoderm forms the dura mater. This distinction is clinically relevant in congenital malformations and tumor origins.

Development of the Ventricular System

The central canal of the neural tube expands and remodels into the ventricular system. The lateral ventricles derive from the telencephalon, the third ventricle from the diencephalon, the cerebral aqueduct from the mesencephalon, and the fourth ventricle from the rhombencephalon. The central canal extends caudally into the spinal cord. Connections include the interventricular foramina linking the lateral ventricles to the third ventricle, the aqueduct connecting the third to the fourth ventricle, and the central canal continuing inferiorly.

Chapter Summary

Neurulation begins in the third week with neural plate formation. Neural folds elevate, converge, and fuse to form the neural tube. Neuropore closure occurs between days twenty-three and twenty-nine; failure leads to neural tube defects. Neural crest cells give rise to diverse structures throughout the body. Brain development proceeds through three- and five-vesicle stages. The meninges arise from neural crest and mesoderm, while the ventricular system derives from the lumen of the neural tube.

Self-Assessment Questions

1. Describe the sequence of events from neural plate formation to neural tube closure.
2. What are the derivatives of neural crest cells?
3. When do the cranial and caudal neuropores close?
4. How does the neural tube differentiate into the major brain vesicles?
5. What are the embryologic origins of the meninges?
6. Which congenital anomalies result from neural tube closure defects?

MCQs

1. Neural crest cells give rise to all of the following EXCEPT:

A. Spinal ganglia
B. Autonomic ganglia
C. Adrenal medulla
D. Cerebral cortex

Answer: D

2. Failure of cranial neuropore closure results in:

A. Spina bifida
B. Anencephaly
C. Hydrocephalus
D. Encephalocele

Answer: B

3. Hirschsprung's disease results from failure of:

A. Neural tube closure
B. Neural crest cell migration
C. Brain vesicle differentiation
D. Spinal cord segmentation

Answer: B

4. Folic acid deficiency is most strongly associated with defects in:
A. Gastrulation
B. Neurulation
C. Implantation
D. Fertilization
E. Organogenesis

Answer: B

CHAPTER VIII

Embryo Folding (Week 4)

Learning Objectives

By the end of this chapter, the student should be able to describe the major morphogenetic events involved in embryo folding, distinguish between cephalic, caudal, and lateral folding, explain how folding transforms the flat trilaminar disc into a cylindrical body form, describe the incorporation of the yolk sac into the embryo and the formation of the primitive gut tube, identify the derivatives of the foregut, midgut, and hindgut, explain the formation of the intraembryonic coelom and its adult derivatives, and recognize clinical correlations associated with abnormalities in folding or ventral body wall formation.

Integrated Video Lecture

Video title: Embryo Folding
Hyperlink: https://youtu.be/rLb19v5Rxok
Source: Private institutional server

Introduction to Embryo Folding

Embryo folding begins at the start of the fourth week and represents a major morphogenetic transformation. The initially flat trilaminar germ disc undergoes coordinated changes that convert it into a three-dimensional cylindrical embryo. Folding is driven by the rapid growth of the ectoderm, especially over the neural tube, differential growth of the embryo relative to the yolk sac, and expansion of the amniotic cavity. Folding occurs simultaneously in three planes: cephalic, caudal, and lateral. These events establish the fundamental body form and initiate organogenesis.

Cephalic Folding

Cephalic folding occurs around days twenty-two to twenty-three, driven by the rapid growth of the cranial neural plate. The neural folds enlarge, and the brain region expands. The septum transversum, primitive heart tube, and oropharyngeal membrane are repositioned ventrally and caudally, relocating the future pericardial cavity to the ventral side of the embryo. This folding places the developing heart and diaphragm into their anatomically correct positions.

Caudal Folding

Caudal folding occurs almost simultaneously with head folding, around day twenty-three. The cloacal membrane shifts ventrally, the connecting stalk moves to the ventral embryonic surface, and the caudal yolk sac region is incorporated into the hindgut. Together, cephalic and caudal folding establish the rostro-caudal orientation of the embryo.

Lateral Folding

Between days twenty-two and twenty-eight, lateral folding results from the rapid growth of the somatic layer of lateral plate mesoderm and the overlying ectoderm. The lateral edges of the embryonic disc move ventrally, and the somatopleure advances toward the midline. Fusion occurs in the ventral midline except at the umbilical region. Lateral folding forms the cylindrical trunk body wall, fuses the ectoderm into a continuous external covering, establishes the intraembryonic coelom, and completes the ventral body wall. Failure of ventral fusion leads to defects such as gastroschisis and omphalocele.

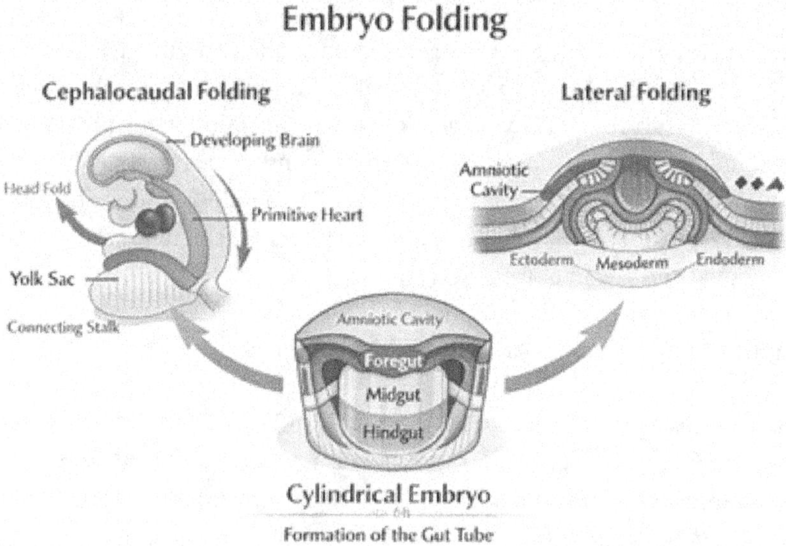

***Embryo Folding**, illustrating both **cephalocaudal** and **lateral folding** that transform the flat trilaminar disc into a cylindrical embryo. It shows the **head and tail folds** bringing the heart and brain into position, while **lateral folds** enclose the yolk sac to form the **gut tube**.*

Formation of the Intraembryonic Coelom

The lateral plate mesoderm splits into somatic (parietal) and splanchnic (visceral) layers. The space between them becomes the intraembryonic coelom, which later partitions into the pericardial, pleural, and peritoneal cavities. Initially continuous, these cavities are separated through subsequent folding and septation.

Incorporation of the Yolk Sac and Formation of the Primitive Gut Tube

Folding incorporates the endoderm-lined yolk sac into the embryo, forming the primitive gut tube. The cranial region of the yolk sac forms the foregut, the caudal region forms the hindgut, and the central region remains temporarily open as the midgut. The midgut retains a connection with the yolk sac via the vitelline duct.

The gut tube is divided into three regions. The **foregut** gives rise to the pharynx, esophagus, stomach, proximal duodenum, liver, gallbladder, pancreas, and respiratory diverticulum. The **midgut** forms the distal duodenum, jejunum, ileum, cecum, appendix, ascending colon, and proximal two-thirds of the transverse colon. The **hindgut** develops into the distal third of the transverse colon, descending and sigmoid colon, rectum, upper anal canal, and cloacal derivatives.

Establishment of Body Cavities and Mesenteries

The primitive gut is anchored to the body wall by mesenteries. The ventral mesentery, present only in the foregut region, gives rise to the lesser Omentum and falciform ligament. The dorsal mesentery extends the length of the gut tube, forming the greater Omentum, mesentery proper, and mesocolon. Organs suspended by mesentery are intraperitoneal, while those pressed against the posterior body wall become secondarily retroperitoneal, such as the pancreas, duodenum, and ascending and descending colon.

Morphogenetic Transformation

Embryo folding converts the flat trilaminar disc into a cylindrical embryo, establishes the ventral body wall, forms the foregut, midgut, and hindgut, creates the intraembryonic coelom, and positions the heart, septum transversum, and cloacal and oropharyngeal membranes correctly. These events also form the primitive umbilical region and set the stage for organogenesis.

Chapter Summary

Embryo folding begins in week four and occurs in cephalic, caudal, and lateral planes. Folding transforms the embryonic disc into a three-dimensional form. Incorporation of the yolk sac results in the primitive gut tube. The intraembryonic coelom forms the major body cavities. Proper folding is essential for closure of the ventral body wall and normal organ positioning.

Self-Assessment Questions

1. What are the three types of embryo folding, and when do they occur?
2. Describe how cephalic and caudal folding reposition early embryonic structures.
3. Explain the formation and significance of the intraembryonic coelom.
4. How does embryo folding contribute to the formation of the primitive gut tube?
5. What are the derivatives of the foregut, midgut, and hindgut?
6. Name two ventral body wall defects resulting from abnormal folding.

MCQs

1. Cephalocaudal folding brings which structures into position?

A. Gut tube and yolk sac
B. Heart and brain
C. Limbs and somites
D. Placenta and membranes

Answer: B

2. Lateral folding is essential for:

A. Formation of the neural tube
B. Closure of the gut tube
C. Development of the placenta
D. Formation of somites

Answer: B

CHAPTER IX

Development of the Placenta (Week 3-20)

Learning Objectives

By the end of this chapter, the student should be able to describe the origin and development of the placenta from fetal and maternal tissues, explain the formation and maturation of chorionic villi and the establishment of uteroplacental circulation, identify the structural features of the mature placenta and their functional significance, outline the metabolic, transport, and endocrine functions of the placenta, describe the embryologic development and structure of the umbilical cord, explain fetal circulation and the function of its major shunts, and recognize major placental anomalies and their clinical implications.

Integrated Video Lecture

Video title: Development of the Placenta
Hyperlink: https://youtu.be/JpQL_xHo2OE
Source: Private institutional server

Introduction and Overview

The placenta is a maternal–fetal organ that forms at the site of blastocyst implantation. The constituents of the Placenta begin to differentiate during week 3 and reach complete structural and vascular maturity by week 20. It serves as the interface for gas exchange, nutrient transfer, waste elimination, and hormone synthesis. Supporting fetal development throughout pregnancy, the placenta is expelled after delivery as the afterbirth. Its functions are metabolic, transport, and endocrine.

Transport and Metabolic Functions

The placenta actively transports essential substances between mother and fetus. Oxygen, glucose, amino acids, fatty acids, vitamins, and trace elements cross from maternal to fetal circulation. IgG antibodies are transferred in the third trimester, conferring passive immunity. Transferrin mediates iron transport, while some medications, toxins, and viral pathogens may also cross. From fetus to mother, carbon dioxide, urea, and other waste products are eliminated. Alpha-fetoprotein, a fetal protein, enters maternal serum and serves as a clinically significant marker.

Endocrine Functions

The placenta secretes hormones essential for pregnancy maintenance, including hCG, human chorionic somatomammotropin (hCS/hPL), progesterone, estrogen, and placental growth hormone. These regulate maternal metabolism, support fetal growth, and maintain uterine quiescence.

Fetal and Maternal Components

The placenta consists of two components: the fetal chorion frondosum and the maternal decidua basalis. Following implantation, the endometrium differentiates into decidua basalis at the implantation site, decidua capsularis covering the conceptus, and decidua parietalis lining the remainder of the uterus.

Development of Chorionic Villi

Villous development proceeds in stages. Primary villi form in week two, composed of cytotrophoblast covered by syncytiotrophoblast. Secondary villi appear in week three as extraembryonic mesoderm invades, forming a mesodermal core. By late week three, tertiary villi develop capillary networks that connect with embryonic vessels in the connecting stalk. Villi near the decidua basalis proliferate to form the chorion frondosum, while those near the decidua capsularis degenerate, forming the chorion laeve. Anchoring villi attach to the decidua basalis, while free villi float in maternal blood and mediate exchange.

Formation of Cotyledons

By weeks fourteen to sixteen, villous invasion of the decidua basalis produces placental septa, dividing the placenta into cotyledons. Each cotyledon contains stem villi and multiple branched villi, forming functional lobules of exchange.

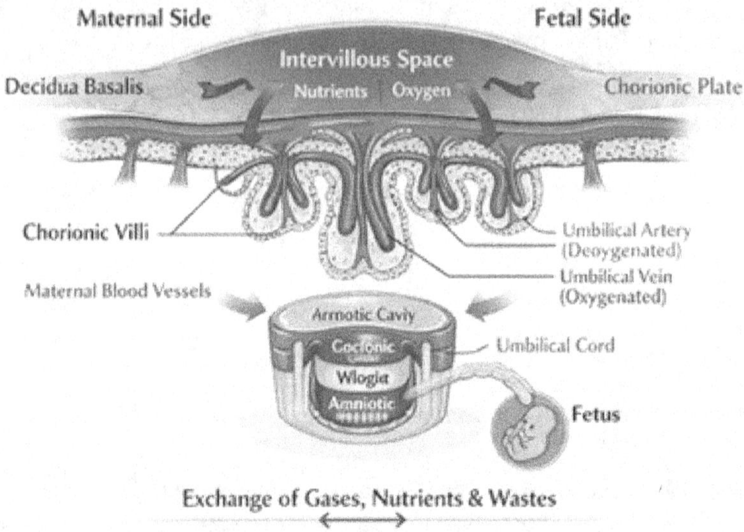

***Development of the Placenta**, showing the structural relationship between the **maternal decidua basalis** and the **fetal chorionic plate**, with chorionic villi extending into the **intervillous space** for maternal–fetal exchange. It depicts the **umbilical arteries and vein**, the **fetal capillaries within villi**, and the **exchange of gases, nutrients, and wastes** across the placental barrier.*

Uteroplacental Circulation

Maternal blood enters the intervillous space via spiral arteries, bathing free villi for gas and nutrient exchange before draining through endometrial veins. Fetal blood arrives via two umbilical arteries, circulates through villous capillaries, and returns oxygenated via the umbilical vein. The placenta acquires complete growth and vascular maturation by week 20 of development.

Structure of the Full-Term Placenta

At term, the placenta is discoid, measuring fifteen to twenty-five centimeters in diameter and weighing approximately five hundred grams.

The fetal surface is smooth, covered by amnion, with the umbilical cord attached centrally. The maternal surface is rough, reddish, and divided into fifteen to twenty cotyledons by decidual septa.

Placental Barrier

In early pregnancy, the barrier consists of syncytiotrophoblast, cytotrophoblast, connective tissue, and capillary endothelium. After week sixteen, cytotrophoblast thins and disappears in many areas, leaving primarily syncytiotrophoblast and capillary endothelium. The barrier is semipermeable, allowing passage of drugs, toxins, and infectious agents, with clinical implications for teratogenicity and fetal infections.

Umbilical Cord Development

The umbilical cord contains two arteries, one vein, Wharton's jelly, and remnants of the allantois and vitelline duct. Early in gestation, it encloses a midgut loop. The cord provides the vital conduit for fetal circulation.

Placental Abnormalities

Placental abruption involves premature separation after twenty weeks, presenting with bleeding and pain. Placenta previa occurs when implantation is in the lower uterine segment, causing painless bleeding in late pregnancy. Placenta accreta spectrum includes abnormal adherence or invasion of the myometrium. Battledore placenta, with marginal cord insertion, is usually incidental but may affect perfusion.

Fetal Circulation

Fetal circulation optimizes oxygen delivery to vital organs. Oxygenated blood travels from the placenta through the umbilical vein, bypasses the liver via the ductus venosus, enters the inferior vena cava, and is shunted through the foramen ovale to the left atrium, then to the brain and upper body. Deoxygenated blood from the superior vena cava enters the right ventricle, passes into the pulmonary artery, and is diverted via the ductus arteriosus to the descending aorta, returning to the placenta through the umbilical arteries. The three major shunts—ductus venosus, foramen ovale, and ductus arteriosus—close at birth to establish adult circulation.

Chapter Summary

The placenta has fetal and maternal components. Chorionic villi progress from primary to tertiary stages, and cotyledons form functional units of exchange. Placental transport includes gases, nutrients, IgG, and selected pathogens. Placental hormones support pregnancy and fetal growth. The placental barrier is semipermeable. The umbilical cord contains two arteries and one vein. Fetal circulation uses three shunts to bypass the lungs. Placental anomalies include previa, abruption, accreta, and cord insertion defects.

Self-Assessment Questions

1. What are the fetal and maternal components of the placenta?
2. Describe the sequence of villous development.
3. What factors cross the placental barrier, and which do not?
4. What are cotyledons, and how do they form?
5. Outline the roles of hCG, progesterone, and estrogen.
6. Describe fetal circulation and identify the three major shunts.
7. What are the clinical consequences of placenta previa and placental abruption?

MCQs

1. Chorionic villi are primarily responsible for:

A. Hormone secretion
B. Maternal–fetal exchange
C. Umbilical cord formation
D. Neural crest migration

Answer: B

2. The maternal contribution to the placenta is:

A. Chorionic plate
B. Decidua basalis
C. Umbilical vein
D. Amnion

Answer: B

CHAPTER X

Development of the Umbilical Cord and Fetal Circulation

Learning Objectives

By the end of this chapter, the student should be able to describe the embryologic origin and structure of the umbilical cord, explain the role of Wharton's jelly and the arrangement of umbilical vessels, outline the pathways of fetal circulation and the function of its major shunts, correlate fetal circulation with placental exchange, and recognize clinical anomalies associated with cord and circulatory development.

Integrated Video Lecture

Video title: Development of the Umbilical Cord and Fetal Circulation
Hyperlink: https://youtu.be/QokrpOAbPyo
Source: Private institutional server

Formation of the Umbilical Cord

The umbilical cord develops from the connecting stalk, yolk sac remnants, and allantois. By the fifth week, the amnion expands and envelops these structures, forming a tubular cord that connects the embryo to the placenta.

Structural Features

- Two umbilical arteries: carry deoxygenated blood from the fetus to the placenta
- One umbilical vein: returns oxygenated blood from the placenta to the fetus
- Wharton's jelly: mucoid connective tissue that cushions and protects vessels
- Vestigial structures: remnants of the allantois and vitelline duct may persist

At term, the cord measures 50–60 cm in length and about 2 cm in diameter, allowing flexibility during fetal movement and delivery.

Fetal Circulation: Overview

Fetal circulation is uniquely adapted to maximize oxygen delivery to vital organs while bypassing nonfunctional fetal lungs. Oxygenated blood from the placenta enters the fetus through the umbilical vein, while deoxygenated blood returns via the umbilical arteries.

Pathways of Oxygenated Blood

1. Oxygenated blood flows from the placenta into the umbilical vein.
2. Most blood bypasses the liver through the **ductus venosus**, entering the inferior vena cava.
3. Blood enters the right atrium, where it is preferentially shunted through the **foramen ovale** into the left atrium.
4. From the left ventricle, blood is pumped into the ascending aorta, supplying the brain and upper body with highly oxygenated blood.

Pathways of Deoxygenated Blood

1. Blood from the superior vena cava enters the right atrium and flows into the right ventricle.
2. It is pumped into the pulmonary artery, but because the lungs are nonfunctional, most blood bypasses them via the **ductus arteriosus**, which connects the pulmonary artery to the descending aorta.
3. Deoxygenated blood then returns to the placenta through the two umbilical arteries.

Major Fetal Shunts

- **Ductus venosus**: bypasses the liver, directing blood into the inferior vena cava
- **Foramen ovale**: shunts blood from the right atrium to the left atrium

- **Ductus arteriosus**: diverts blood from the pulmonary artery to the descending aorta

These shunts ensure efficient distribution of oxygenated blood to the brain and myocardium. At birth, they close functionally and structurally, establishing adult circulation.

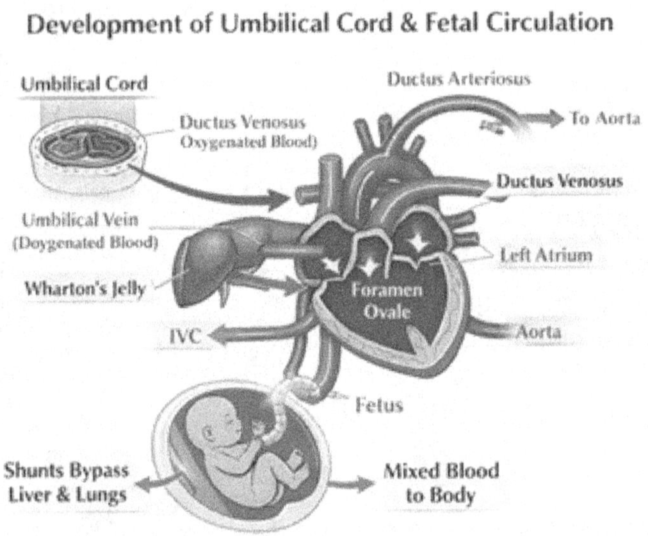

Development of the Umbilical Cord and Fetal Circulation, showing the structural and functional relationships between the umbilical vessels, Wharton's jelly, and the three major fetal shunts — ductus venosus, foramen ovale, and ductus arteriosus.

Clinical Correlations

- **Single umbilical artery**: associated with congenital anomalies of the cardiovascular and urogenital systems
- **Patent ductus arteriosus (PDA)**: persistence of the ductus arteriosus after birth, leading to abnormal circulation

- **Short or excessively long cords**: may cause complications during delivery, including cord prolapse or entanglement
- **True knots or velamentous insertion**: may impair blood flow and compromise fetal oxygenation

Chapter Summary

The umbilical cord develops from the connecting stalk and contains two arteries, one vein, and Wharton's jelly. Fetal circulation is adapted to bypass the lungs and liver, using three major shunts: ductus venosus, foramen ovale, and ductus arteriosus. These pathways ensure optimal oxygen delivery to vital organs. At birth, closure of the shunts establishes adult circulation. Clinical anomalies of the cord or shunts can significantly impact fetal and neonatal outcomes.

Self-Assessment Questions

1. What are the structural components of the umbilical cord?
2. Describe the pathway of oxygenated blood from the placenta to the fetal brain.
3. What are the functions of the ductus venosus, foramen ovale, and ductus arteriosus?
4. How does fetal circulation differ from postnatal circulation?
5. What clinical anomalies are associated with the umbilical cord and fetal shunt to

MCQs

1. The ductus venosus allows blood to bypass the:

A.Lungs
B. Liver
C. Kidneys
D. Heart

Answer: B

2. The foramen ovale shunts blood from:

A. Right atrium to left atrium
B. Right ventricle to left ventricle
C. Pulmonary artery to aorta
D. Umbilical vein to inferior vena cava

Answer: A

3. The umbilical vein carries:

A. Deoxygenated blood to the placenta
B. Oxygenated blood to the fetus
C. Mixed blood to liver
D. Blood to lungs
E. Blood to heart only

Answer: B

Part II – Systemic Development

CHAPTER XI

Development of the Heart

Learning objectives

By the end of this chapter, the student should be able to describe the early formation of the cardiogenic region and the paired endocardial tubes, explain the successive morphogenetic events: heart tube formation, looping, and temporalization, outline the embryologic origins of major cardiac components (atria, ventricles, outflow tracts), describe the processes of atrial, ventricular, and outflow tract septation and valve formation, recognize the embryologic basis, pathophysiology, and typical clinical features of common congenital heart defects (ASD, VSD, PDA, tetralogy of Fallot, truncus arteriosus, transposition), and apply embryologic knowledge to basic diagnostic reasoning (e.g., why right-to-left vs left-to-right shunts occur; basics of Eisenmenger physiology).

Integrated Video Lecture
Video title: Development of the Heart
Hyperlink: https://www.youtube.com/watch?v=KFADbUEigM0
Source: Private institutional server

Overview and clinical relevance

Congenital heart disease affects approximately 1–2% of live births and is a leading cause of neonatal morbidity. Understanding cardiac embryology clarifies the origins of structural defects, their haemodynamic consequences, and the rationale for many diagnostic and surgical strategies.

Cardiac morphogenesis begins in the **third week** and proceeds through a coordinated sequence of specification, tube formation, looping, septation, and remodeling.

Cardiogenic region and heart tube formation

- The cardiogenic region arises from splanchnic (splanchnopleuric) mesoderm in a horseshoe-shaped area cranial to the neural plate. Signals from adjacent endoderm induce cardiac differentiation.
- Endothelial precursors coalesce to form paired endocardial tubes by ~day 19–20.
- Fusion of the tubes in the midline generates a single primitive heart tube, invested externally by myocardium (from splanchnic mesoderm) and separated from the pericardial cavity by the intraembryonic coelom.

Five early dilatations of the linear heart tube

(from cranial to caudal):

1. Truncus arteriosus
2. Bulbus cordis
3. Primitive ventricle
4. Primitive atrium
5. Sinus venosus

These regions are precursors of the definitive outflow tracts, ventricles, atria, and venous inflow.

Cardiac looping and positional changes

- Rapid growth of the heart tube causes rightward (dextral) looping (bulboventricular loop), repositioning the future chambers: the bulbus cordis moves antero-inferiorly; the primitive ventricle moves anteriorly/left; the atrium shifts posteriorly/superiorly; the sinus venosus becomes posterior.
- Looping establishes the basic ventricular and atrial relationships required for later septation and alignment of inflow and outflow tracts.

Septation of the heart

Atrioventricular canal & endocardial cushions

- Endocardial cushions form in the atrioventricular canal and conotruncal region from local mesenchyme and endocardial-to-mesenchyme transformation. Fusion of dorsal and ventral AV cushions partitions the common AV canal into right and left AV orifices and contributes to valve formation (mitral and tricuspid valves).

Atrial septation

- **Septum primum** grows from the roof toward the AV cushions, leaving the **ostium primum**, which later closes. Apoptosis in the upper septum primum creates the **ostium secundum**.
- **Septum secundum** forms to the right of the septum primum, leaving a foramen ovale. In fetal life, right-to-left shunting occurs through the foramen ovale; after birth, rising left atrial pressure functionally closes it, and anatomical fusion usually follows to form the fossa ovalis.

Ventricular septation

- The muscular interventricular septum grows upward from the floor of the primitive ventricle toward the AV cushions. A small **interventricular foramen** remains and is closed by the membranous septum formation from contributions of endocardial cushions and conotruncal ridges (involving neural crest cells). Failure of these elements to fuse produces membranous ventricular septal defects (VSDs).

Outflow tract (conotruncal) septation

- Conotruncal (truncal and bulbar) ridges grow and spiral to form the **aorticopulmonary (spiral) septum**, dividing the outflow tract into the ascending aorta and pulmonary trunk. Neural crest cells contribute critically to this process. Abnormal neural crest migration or conotruncal septation leads to outflow tract anomalies (e.g., persistent truncus arteriosus, transposition of the great arteries, tetralogy of Fallot).

Valve formation and ventricular remodeling

- Valve leaflets arise from endocardial cushion tissue with shaping by blood flow and myocardial signaling.
- The bulbus cordis and truncus contribute to the smooth outflow tracts: the bulbus cordis contributes to the right ventricular outflow (conus arteriosus) and left ventricular outflow (aortic vestibule).
- Trabeculated parts of ventricles derive from the primitive ventricular cavity.

Embryologic origins of specific cardiac regions (summary)

- Right ventricle (trabeculated portion): primitive ventricle
- Left ventricle (trabeculated portion): primitive ventricle
- Outflow tracts (proximal): bulbus cordis / truncus arteriosus → partitioned by spiral septum
- Atria: primitive atrium (trabeculated) + incorporation of sinus venosus parts (smooth walls)
- Sinoatrial and venous components: derivatives of sinus venosus (right horn → sinus venarum; left horn → coronary sinus

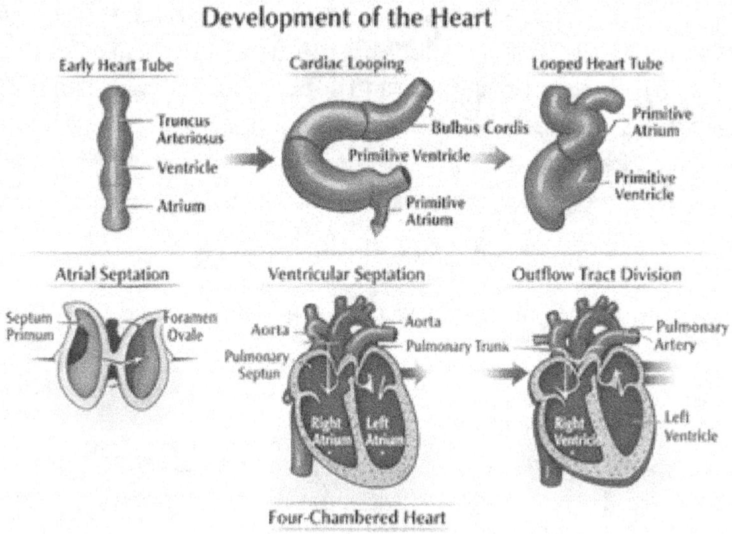

Development of the Heart, illustrating the transformation from the ***primitive heart tube*** *to the* ***four-chambered heart****. It traces the sequence of* ***heart tube formation, looping, septation, and outflow tract division****, showing how the* ***truncus arteriosus, bulbus cordis, primitive ventricle, and atrium*** *reorganize into the mature cardiac structure. The lower panels highlight* ***atrial and ventricular septation*** *and the* ***aorticopulmonary septum****, culminating in the fully formed heart with distinct oxygenated and deoxygenated pathways.*

Common congenital cardiac anomalies.
Embryologic Basis, Pathophysiology, and Clinical Features

The following concise summaries replace the informal and speculative passages in the transcript and present clinically useful, exam-relevant material.

Ventricular septal defect (VSD)

- **Embryology:** Failure of the membranous septum closure (most common) or muscular septal defects due to incomplete muscular septum formation. Membranous VSDs arise from defective fusion of the muscular septum with endocardial cushions and conotruncal ridges.

- **Hemodynamic:** Left-to-right shunt causes volume overload of pulmonary circulation and left heart; large defects may progress to pulmonary overcirculation and pulmonary vascular disease (Eisenmenger physiology) with reversal to right-to-left shunt.
- **Clinical:** Harsh holosystolic murmur if small; large defects cause heart failure, poor feeding in infants, and recurrent pulmonary infections.

Atrial septal defect (ASD) — secundum type (foramen secundum)

- **Embryology:** Excessive resorption of septum primum or deficient growth of septum secundum.
- **Hemodynamic:** Chronic left-to-right shunt at atrial level → right atrial/ ventricular dilation, paradoxical emboli risk, eventual pulmonary vascular disease if large.
- **Clinical:** Fixed, widely split S2; may be asymptomatic in childhood.

Patent ductus arteriosus (PDA)

- **Embryology/physiology:** Ductus arteriosus connects pulmonary artery to descending aorta in fetal life; patency is maintained by low oxygen tension and circulating prostaglandins (notably PGE2). After birth, increased P_{aO_2} and a decline in prostaglandins promote functional closure; permanent anatomical closure follows.
- **Pathology:** Persistent PDA → continuous machinery murmur, left heart volume overload, pulmonary overcirculation.
- **Management note:** Pharmacologic closure uses NSAIDs (indomethacin/ ibuprofen) to inhibit prostaglandin synthesis; prostaglandin E analogs (e.g., alprostadil) are used to maintain ductal patency when needed in cyanotic duct-dependent lesions.

Tetralogy of Fallot (TOF)

- **Embryology:** Anterosuperior displacement of the conotruncal (infundibular) septum due to abnormal neural crest migration results in four features:

1. **Pulmonary stenosis** (right ventricular outflow obstruction)
2. **Ventricular septal defect** (usually membranous)
3. **Overriding aorta** (aorta receives blood from both ventricles)
4. **Right ventricular hypertrophy** (secondary to outflow obstruction)

- **Hemodynamic & clinical:** Right-to-left shunt severity determines cyanosis; "Tet Spells" (hypercyanotic episodes) can occur; management is surgical.

Persistent truncus arteriosus

- **Embryology:** Failure of conotruncal ridges to form or to spiral and fuse results in a single arterial trunk supplying the systemic, pulmonary, and coronary circulations.
- **Clinical:** Early heart failure, cyanosis; requires corrective surgery.

Transposition of the great arteries (TGA)

- **Embryology:** Failure of the aorticopulmonary septum to spiral results in parallel rather than crossed outflow tracts (aorta from right ventricle; pulmonary artery from left ventricle).
- **Clinical:** Severe cyanosis at birth unless mixing occurs (ASD, VSD, PDA); early prostaglandin infusion (to keep ductus arteriosus open) and surgical repair are typically required.

Tricuspid atresia and Ebstein anomaly (selected right-heart lesions)

- **Tricuspid atresia:** Absence of tricuspid valve → hypoplastic right ventricle; requires interatrial communication and PDA for pulmonary blood flow.
- **Ebstein anomaly:** Downward displacement of tricuspid valve leaflets → atrialization of right ventricle; associated with tricuspid regurgitation and arrhythmias; classic association with maternal lithium exposure

(historically reported).

Coarctation of the aorta

- **Embryology:** Abnormal development of the aortic arch/descending aorta (postductal or preductal types); pathogenesis includes abnormal flow and possibly migration anomalies.
- **Clinical:** Differential blood pressures (upper > lower extremities), late hypertension, claudication; associated with bicuspid aortic valve.

Eisenmenger physiology (brief)

- Chronic, large **left-to-right shunts** (e.g., large VSD, ASD, PDA) can cause progressive pulmonary vascular remodeling and pulmonary hypertension. When pulmonary vascular resistance exceeds systemic resistance, shunt reverses to **right-to-left**, producing cyanosis, clubbing, and systemic hypoxemia (Eisenmenger syndrome). Reversal is typically irreversible; management focuses on preventing pulmonary vascular disease and on advanced therapies when appropriate.

Clinical and diagnostic correlations

- **Prenatal ultrasound** can detect many major structural defects (e.g., conotruncal anomalies, hypoplastic left heart, large VSDs) in the second trimester; fetal echocardiography is diagnostic.
- **Biochemical and genetic** associations: certain teratogens (e.g., isotretinoin), maternal diabetes, chromosomal anomalies (e.g., trisomy 21 associated with endocardial cushion defects) increase the risk.
- **Medical management:** prostaglandin E1 to maintain ductal patency in duct-dependent lesions; diuretics/afterload reduction for heart failure; definitive management is often surgical repair.

Chapter summary

- The heart develops from a midline tube derived from splanchnic mesoderm; subsequent looping and septation generate chambers and separate outflow tracts.
- Endocardial cushions, conotruncal ridges (neural crest dependent), and muscular growth coordinate the formation of septa and valves.
- Most congenital cardiac defects have clear embryologic correlates: failure of fusion (VSD), abnormal conotruncal septation (TOF, TGA, truncus), and valve/atrioventricular anomalies (endocardial cushion defects).
- Hemodynamic consequences determine clinical presentation and timing of symptoms; early recognition and appropriate intervention significantly improve outcomes.

Self-assessment questions

1. List the five early dilatations of the primitive heart tube and name their principal adult derivatives.
2. Explain how abnormal neural crest migration contributes to tetralogy of Fallot and truncus arteriosus.
3. Differentiate membranous and muscular VSD embryologically and describe the clinical consequences of a large VSD.
4. Why does a patent ductus arteriosus produce a continuous "machinery" murmur? How is PDA medically closed?
5. Describe the embryologic mechanism that produces transposition of the great arteries.

MCQs

1. The primitive heart tube is formed by fusion of:

A. Neural crest cells
B. Endocardial tubes
C. Mesonephric ducts
D.Somites

Answer: B

2. Abnormal looping of the heart tube can result in:

A.Tetralogy of Fallot
B. Transposition of great vessels
C. Patent ductus arteriosus
D. Atrial septal defect

Answer: B

3. Failure of neural crest cell migration can lead to:

A. ASD
B. VSD
C. Tetralogy of Fallot
D. PDA
E. Coarctation

Answer: C

4. The foramen ovale allows blood flow between:

A. RA → RV
B. RA → LA
C. LA → LV
D. RV → pulmonary artery
E. Aorta → pulmonary artery

Answer: B

CHAPTER XII

Development of the Pharyngeal Arches (Week 4)

Learning Objectives

By the end of this chapter, the student should be able to describe the structure and organization of the pharyngeal apparatus, identify the derivatives of each pharyngeal arch, pouch, groove, and membrane, explain the contributions of neural crest cells to craniofacial development, understand the embryologic basis of key clinical conditions such as DiGeorge syndrome and branchial cysts/fistulas, and integrate arch derivatives with their associated cranial nerves, muscles, skeletal elements, and arterial components.

Integrated Video Lecture

Video Title: Development of the Pharyngeal Arches
Hyperlink: https://youtu.be/IgW7Qq47F3A
Source: Private institutional server

Overview of the Pharyngeal Apparatus

Beginning in the fourth week, a series of paired mesenchymal swellings appear on the ventrolateral surface of the developing head and neck. Collectively, these structures form the pharyngeal apparatus, composed of arches, pouches, grooves, and membranes.

Each pharyngeal arch contains a cartilaginous bar, a cranial nerve, skeletal muscle components, an arterial element, and migratory neural crest cells. In humans, five functional arches are present: arches 1, 2, 3, 4, and 6. The fifth arch is rudimentary and regresses quickly, while the sixth arch is present but not externally visible.

Pharyngeal Grooves, Pouches, and Membranes

Pharyngeal grooves (clefts) are ectoderm-lined depressions between arches externally. Pharyngeal pouches are endoderm-lined outpocketings of the foregut internally. Pharyngeal membranes are regions where ectoderm and endoderm come into direct contact, separated only by thin mesenchyme. Of these, only membrane 1 persists in the adult as the tympanic membrane.

Derivatives of the Pharyngeal Arches

First Arch (Mandibular Arch)

- Nerve: CN V3 (mandibular division of trigeminal)
- Skeletal derivatives: maxilla, zygomatic bone, squamous temporal bone, mandible (via Meckel's cartilage), malleus, incus, sphenomandibular ligament
- Muscles: mastication, mylohyoid, anterior belly of digastric, tensor tympani, tensor veli palatini
- Artery: maxillary artery
- Associated structures: groove 1 → external acoustic meatus; pouch 1 → auditory tube and middle ear cavity; membrane 1 → tympanic membrane

Second Arch (Hyoid Arch)

- Nerve: CN VII (facial nerve)
- Skeletal derivatives: stapes, styloid process, stylohyoid ligament, lesser horn and upper body of hyoid
- Muscles: facial expression, posterior belly of digastric, stylohyoid, stapedius
- Artery: stapedial artery (embryonic, regresses)
- Pouch: palatine tonsil
- Grooves 2–4: form cervical sinus, later obliterated

Third Arch

- Nerve: CN IX (glossopharyngeal)
- Skeletal derivatives: greater horn and lower body of the hyoid
- Muscle: stylopharyngeus
- Arteries: common carotid, proximal internal carotid

- Pouch: dorsal wing → inferior parathyroid; ventral wing → thymus

Fourth Arch

- Nerve: CN X (superior laryngeal branch)
- Skeletal derivatives: thyroid, cricoid, corniculate, cuneiform cartilages
- Muscles: pharyngeal constrictors (except stylopharyngeus), cricothyroid, soft palate muscles (except tensor Veli palatini)
- Arteries: right subclavian (proximal), arch of aorta (left)
- Pouch: dorsal wing → superior parathyroid; ventral wing → ultimobranchial body (C-cells of thyroid)

Sixth Arch

- Nerve: CN X (recurrent laryngeal branch)
- Skeletal derivatives: laryngeal cartilages (arytenoid, cricoid, corniculate, cuneiform)
- Muscles: intrinsic laryngeal muscles (except cricothyroid), striated muscles of the upper esophagus
- Arteries: proximal pulmonary artery (right), ductus arteriosus (left)

Neural Crest Cells and Craniofacial Patterning

Neural crest cells migrate extensively into the pharyngeal arches, contributing to Viscerocranial bones and cartilage, sensory ganglia, cardiac outflow tract septation, connective tissue of the face and neck, and odontoblasts. Abnormal migration or differentiation leads to craniofacial anomalies and conotruncal cardiac defects.

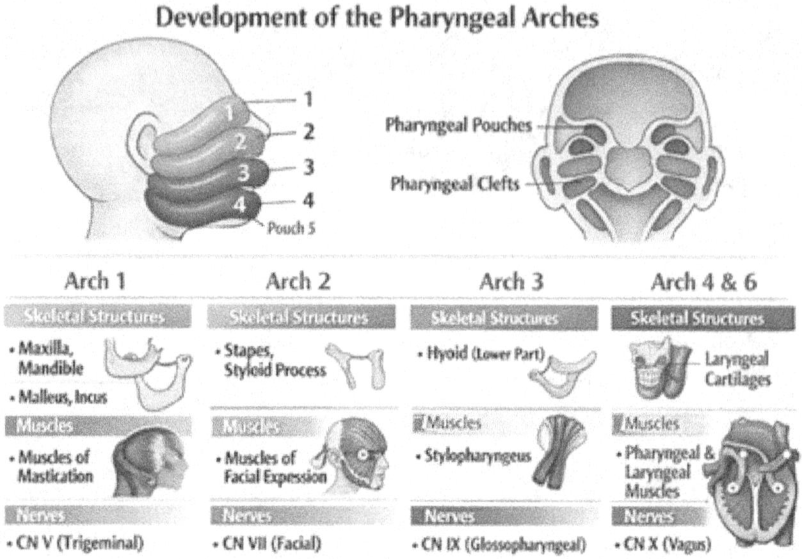

***Development of the Pharyngeal Arches**, showing the five arches and their derivatives in skeletal, muscular, and neural components. It depicts the **lateral and cross-sectional views** of the embryonic head with labeled **arches, pouches, and clefts**, followed by a structured table of derivatives:*

- ***Arch 1:** Maxilla, mandible, muscles of mastication, CN V.*
- ***Arch 2:** Stapes, styloid process, muscles of facial expression, CN VII.*
- ***Arch 3:** Lower hyoid, stylopharyngeus, CN IX.*
- ***Arch 4 & 6:** Laryngeal cartilages, pharyngeal and laryngeal muscles, CN X.*

Clinical Correlations

DiGeorge Syndrome (22q11.2 deletion)

Failure of development of the third and fourth pouches results in thymic aplasia, hypocalcemia due to parathyroid deficiency, conotruncal cardiac defects, and craniofacial anomalies.

Branchial Cysts and Fistulas

Failure of cervical sinus obliteration produces branchial cysts along the anterior border of the sternocleidomastoid. Persistence of both pouch and groove leads to branchial fistulas, forming tracts between the pharynx and skin.

Integrated Summary Table

Arch	Cartilage	Muscles	Nerve	Artery
1	Maxilla, mandible, malleus, incus	Mastication, mylohyoid, ant. digastric, tensors	CN V3	Maxillary artery
2	Stapes, styloid process, lesser hyoid	Facial expression, post. digastric, stylohyoid, stapedius	CN VII	Stapedial artery
3	Greater horn + lower hyoid	Stylopharyngeus	CN IX	Common + proximal internal carotid
4	Thyroid, cricoid, pharyngeal cartilages	Cricothyroid, pharyngeal constrictors, soft palate	CN X (SLN)	Arch of aorta (L), right subclavian (R)
6	Laryngeal cartilages	Intrinsic laryngeal (except cricothyroid), upper esophagus	CN X (RLN)	Ductus arteriosus (L), pulmonary artery (R)

Chapter Summary

The pharyngeal arches form key components of the face, neck, larynx, and upper thorax. Each arch contains specific muscle, cartilage, arterial, and cranial nerve elements. Pouches and grooves form internal and external structures, most of which regress except those of the first arch. Neural crest migration is essential for craniofacial and cardiac development. DiGeorge syndrome and branchial cysts/fistulas exemplify anomalies of pharyngeal development.

Self-Assessment Questions

1. What are the major derivatives of the first pharyngeal arch?
2. Which pharyngeal pouch gives rise to the thymus and inferior parathyroid glands?
3. What is the embryologic origin of the tympanic membrane?
4. Why do branchial cysts occur along the anterior border of the sternocleidomastoid?

5. Explain the embryologic basis of conotruncal defects in DiGeorge syndrome.
6. Which arch derivatives fail to form when the recurrent laryngeal nerve is damaged?

MCQs

1. A child has a cyst along the anterior border of the sternocleidomastoid muscle. This is most likely derived from:

A. First branchial cleft
B. Second branchial cleft
C. Third branchial cleft
D. Fourth pouch
E. Neural crest

Answer: B

2. The thymus develops from which structure?

A. First pouch
B. Second pouch
C. Third pouch
D. Fourth pouch
E. Fifth arch

Answer: C

3. The first pharyngeal arch gives rise to:

A. Maxilla and mandible
B. Stapes and styloid process
C. Laryngeal cartilage
D. Stylopharyngeus muscle

Answer: A

4. The nerve associated with the second pharyngeal arch is:

A.CN V
B.CN VII
C.CN IX
D.CN X

Answer: B

CHAPTER XIII

Development of the Gastrointestinal Tract

Learning Objectives

By the end of this chapter, the student should be able to describe the origin of the primitive gut tube following embryo folding, identify the adult derivatives of the foregut, midgut, and hindgut, explain the development of the esophagus, stomach, duodenum, liver, biliary tree, pancreas, and spleen, describe midgut rotation and physiological umbilical herniation, outline the partitioning of the cloaca by the Urorectal septum, and recognize major congenital anomalies including Esophageal atresia, pyloric stenosis, duodenal atresia, annular pancreas, malrotation, Meckel diverticulum, omphalocele, volvulus, and imperforate anus.

Integrated Video Lecture
Video Title: Development of the Gastrointestinal Tract
Hyperlink: https://youtu.be/8fhDY1VbeRw
Source: Private institutional server

Section 1 — Formation of the Primitive Gut Tube

Gut development begins in the **fourth week**, as **cranial–caudal** and **lateral folding** convert the flat trilaminar embryo into a cylindrical form. This folding incorporates part of the **endoderm-lined yolk sac** into the embryo to form the **primitive gut tube**, which remains temporarily connected to the residual yolk sac by the **vitelline duct**.

The primitive gut tube is classically divided into:

- **Foregut**
- **Midgut**
- **Hindgut**

The foregut and hindgut end blindly at the Anterior intestinal portal (foregut) and the Posterior intestinal portal (hindgut). The midgut remains temporarily open to the yolk sac.

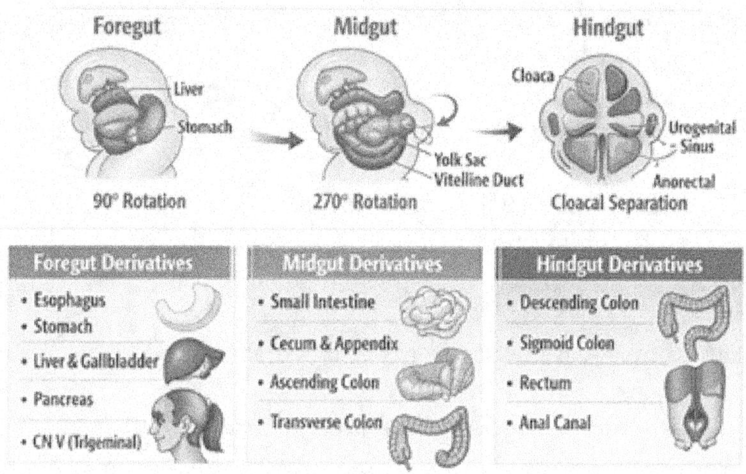

This diagram illustrates the origin of the gastrointestinal tract from the endodermal gut tube. The foregut gives rise to the pharynx, esophagus, stomach, and proximal duodenum, while the midgut forms the distal duodenum, small intestine, and part of the colon. The hindgut contributes to the remainder of the colon and rectum. Intestinal rotation and fixation establish the definitive abdominal arrangement, with the midgut undergoing characteristic herniation and return. Disruptions in these processes can result in malrotation or congenital anomalies such as Meckel's diverticulum.

Endodermal and Mesodermal Contributions

- **Endoderm** gives rise to:
    - mucosal epithelium
    - submucosal glands
    - epithelial lining of liver, gallbladder, pancreas, and intrahepatic biliary tree
- **Visceral mesoderm** forms:

  - lamina propria
  - muscularis mucosa
  - submucosa and connective tissue
  - muscularis externa
  - adventitia and serosa

- **Neural crest cells** migrate into the gut wall to form:
  - **Myenteric (Auerbach)** and **submucosal (Meissner)** plexuses
  - Essential for intestinal motility

(Hirschsprung disease results from failed neural crest migration.)

Section 2 Mesenteries and Body Cavities

The primitive gut tube is suspended by:

1. **Dorsal mesentery**

- Extends the entire length of the tube
- Later forms: mesentery proper, greater Omentum, mesocolon

2. **Ventral mesentery**

- Exists only in the foregut region
- Derivatives:
  - **Falciform ligament**
  - **Lesser Omentum**

The **septum transversum**, originally cranial to the heart, moves caudally during folding and gives rise to:

- central tendon of the diaphragm
- hepatic stroma / connective tissue
- hepatic stellate cells
- hemopoietic tissue precursors

Section 3 Foregut Development

Foregut derivatives include:

- Pharynx, Esophagus
- Stomach, proximal duodenum
- Liver, biliary apparatus
- Pancreas
- Spleen (mesodermal organ associated with the foregut)

Development of the Esophagus

- Originates from the foregut distal to the pharynx.
- **The tracheoesophageal septum** separates the Esophagus from the tracheobronchial diverticulum.
- Endoderm initially proliferates and **temporarily occludes the lumen**; later **recanalization** restores patency.
- **Upper one-third muscle** → derived from **pharyngeal arch mesoderm → striated muscle.**
- **Lower two-thirds** → smooth muscle from splanchnic mesoderm.

Clinical correlation:

- **Esophageal atresia + tracheoesophageal fistula** result from abnormal partitioning by the tracheoesophageal septum.

Development of the Stomach

Dilation and rotation

- Appears during week 4 as a fusiform dilation of the foregut.
- Rotates **90° clockwise** around its longitudinal axis:

- left side → anterior
- right side → posterior

- Dorsal border grows faster → **greater curvature**
- Ventral border → **lesser curvature**

Muscular development

- Smooth muscle layers appear in week 5 from splanchnic mesoderm.

Clinical correlation:

- **Hypertrophic pyloric stenosis**
    - Hypertrophy of pyloric circular muscle → projectile, non-bilious vomiting at ~3–4 weeks.

Dorsal and Ventral Mesogastrium: Omenta and Spleen

Dorsal mesogastrium

- Elongates and is pulled leftward → **lesser sac (omental bursa)**
- Forms the **greater Omentum** (double-layered apron)

Spleen

- Develops in the dorsal mesogastrium (week 5) from **mesenchymal condensations**
- Fetal spleen is lobulated; lobules regress before birth
- Forms ligaments:

  - Gastrosplenic
  - Lienorenal

Ventral mesogastrium

- Contains the **liver bud** → forms the falciform ligament and lesser Omentum

Liver and Extrahepatic Biliary System

Arise from the hepatic diverticulum (week 4).

Hepatic diverticulum divides into:

- Cranial portion → liver parenchyma (hepatocytes)
- Caudal portion → gallbladder + cystic duct

Endoderm forms:

- Hepatocytes
- Epithelial lining of the biliary tree

Mesoderm (septum transversum) forms:

- Connective tissue
- Kupffer cells
- Hemopoietic tissue

Pancreas

Develops from two buds:

- **Dorsal pancreatic bud** (larger)

- **Ventral pancreatic bud** (near bile duct)

Rotation of the duodenum brings the ventral bud dorsally → **fusion** of buds.

Derivatives

- **Ventral bud** → uncinate process + inferior head
- **Dorsal bud** → remainder of pancreas
- **Main pancreatic duct** = ventral duct + distal dorsal duct

Clinical correlation:

- **Annular pancreas**
  - Ventral bud encircles duodenum → obstruction, bilious vomiting.

Section 4 Midgut Development

Midgut derivatives:

- Distal duodenum
- Jejunum and ileum
- Cecum and appendix
- Ascending colon
- Proximal two-thirds of the transverse colon

Physiological Umbilical Herniation (Week 6)

- Midgut forms a **U-shaped loop** and herniates into the umbilical cord due to limited abdominal space (large liver, kidneys, rapid growth).
- Loop rotates **90° counterclockwise** around the superior mesenteric artery (SMA).

Return to the Abdomen (Week 10)

- Midgut returns to the abdominal cavity.
- Undergoes additional 180° counterclockwise rotation (total = 270°).

Final positions

- Jejunum → left upper quadrant
- Ileum → central and right regions
- Cecum migrates to the right iliac fossa

Retroperitoneal fixation

- Ascending and descending colon fuse to the posterior abdominal wall → secondarily retroperitoneal.

Clinical Correlations of Midgut Development

Malrotation

- Cecum remains high → predisposes to **volvulus**, bilious vomiting.

Omphalocele

- Failure of the midgut to return → abdominal contents herniated into the umbilical cord, covered by amniotic membrane.

Meckel Diverticulum

Persistence of the **vitelline duct** → true diverticulum on the ileum.

Rule of 2s:

- 2% population
- 2 feet from the ileocecal valve
- 2 inches long
- may contain gastric or pancreatic mucosa
- presents before age 2

Section 5 Hindgut Development

Hindgut derivatives:

- Distal third of the transverse colon
- Descending colon
- Sigmoid colon
- Rectum
- Upper anal canal
- Cloaca and derivatives
- Portions of the bladder and urethra

Retroperitonealization

- Descending colon → secondarily retroperitoneal
- Sigmoid mesentery persists

Section 6 — Cloacal Division and Anal Canal Development Cloaca

A common chamber receiving:

- hindgut
- allantois
- mesonephric ducts

Urorectal septum (Week 4–7)

- Mesodermal septum grows caudally
- Divides the cloaca into:
    - Dorsal anorectal canal
    - Ventral urogenital sinus

Membrane rupture (Week 7)

- Anal membrane → anal orifice
- Urogenital membrane → urogenital opening

Anal canal origins

- Upper 2/3 → endoderm (hindgut)
- Lower 1/3 → ectoderm (proctodeum)

Pectinate line marks this junction.

Clinical Correlation: Anorectal Malformations

Arise from abnormal cloacal partitioning or membrane rupture. Spectrum includes:

- Imperforate anus
- Anal stenosis
- Rectourethral fistula (boys)
- Rectovaginal fistula (girls)
- Cloacal malformations

Often associated with vertebral, cardiac, renal, or limb anomalies (VACTERL association).

Chapter Summary

- Embryo folding incorporates endoderm into the primitive gut tube.
- Foregut gives rise to the Esophagus, stomach, proximal duodenum, liver, biliary tree, pancreas, and spleen.
- Midgut herniates, rotates 270°, and forms the jejunum, ileum, cecum, and proximal colon.
- Hindgut forms the distal colon, rectum, part of the bladder, and anal canal.
- Recanalization defects cause atresias; rotation defects cause malrotation and volvulus; vitelline duct remnants cause Meckel diverticulum.
- Cloacal partitioning forms anorectal and urogenital tracts; errors produce anorectal malformations.

Self-Assessment Questions

1. Which germ layers contribute to the mucosal epithelium and muscular layers of the gut?
2. Describe the developmental rotations that form the definitive stomach shape.
3. What are the derivatives of the dorsal and ventral pancreatic buds?
4. Explain the steps of midgut rotation and physiological herniation.
5. What is the embryologic basis of Meckel diverticulum?
6. How does the Urorectal septum contribute to anorectal development?
7. What developmental anomalies result from failure of duodenal recanalization?

MCQs

1. The midgut undergoes a characteristic rotation of:

A. 90° clockwise
B. 180° clockwise
C. 270° counterclockwise

D. 360° counterclockwise

Answer: C

2. Meckel's diverticulum results from persistence of the:

A. Thyroglossal duct
B. Vitelline duct
C. Urachus
D. Allantois

Answer: B

CHAPTER XIV

Development of the Respiratory System

Learning Objectives

By the end of this chapter, the student should be able to describe the origin of the respiratory diverticulum from the foregut, explain the formation of the larynx, trachea, bronchi, and lungs, identify the four histologic stages of lung development and their clinical significance, describe the genetic and molecular signals that regulate early lung specification, understand the causes and embryologic basis of tracheoesophageal fistulas and Esophageal atresia, and explain the role of surfactant in neonatal respiratory physiology.

Integrated Video Lecture

Video Title: Development of the Respiratory System
Hyperlink: https://youtu.be/EPR_OXlVhRs
Source: Private institutional server

Embryologic Origins

The respiratory system begins in week four as an endodermal outgrowth from the primitive foregut, called the laryngotracheal diverticulum. Endoderm forms the epithelial lining of the larynx, trachea, bronchi, bronchioles, and alveoli, while splanchnic mesoderm contributes cartilage, smooth muscle, connective tissue, and visceral pleura. This illustrates the essential endoderm–mesoderm interaction in organogenesis.

Molecular Regulation

Retinoic acid from mesoderm induces foregut endoderm to express TBX4, initiating lung budding and tracheoesophageal separation. FGF10 from splanchnic mesoderm promotes branching morphogenesis. Disruption of these signals results in incomplete lung development, tracheoesophageal anomalies, or hypoplastic lungs.

Tracheoesophageal Separation

The respiratory diverticulum enlarges ventrally, while the dorsal foregut remains the esophagus. A longitudinal tracheoesophageal septum separates the two. Ventral derivatives include the larynx, trachea, and bronchial tree; dorsal derivatives form the esophagus. Abnormal partitioning produces Esophageal atresia and tracheoesophageal fistula.

Development of the Larynx

Endoderm forms the epithelium and glands, while cartilage and muscles derive from the fourth and sixth pharyngeal arches. Innervation is via the superior laryngeal nerve (arch 4) and the recurrent laryngeal nerve (arch 6). Between weeks seven and ten, epithelial proliferation temporarily occludes the lumen; recanalization restores patency, forming ventricles and vocal folds. Failure of recanalization causes laryngeal atresia.

Development of the Trachea

Endoderm forms the epithelium and glands, while splanchnic mesoderm produces smooth muscle and C-shaped cartilage rings. The trachea remains midline as the bronchi branch asymmetrically.

Development of Bronchi and Lungs

By week five, the lung bud bifurcates into right and left primary bronchi. Secondary bronchi form by week six to seven (three on the right, two on the left). Tertiary bronchi develop thereafter, establishing bronchopulmonary segments. By week twenty-four, approximately fourteen generations of branching have occurred. Surrounding mesenchyme forms cartilage, smooth muscle, connective tissue, and vascular networks.

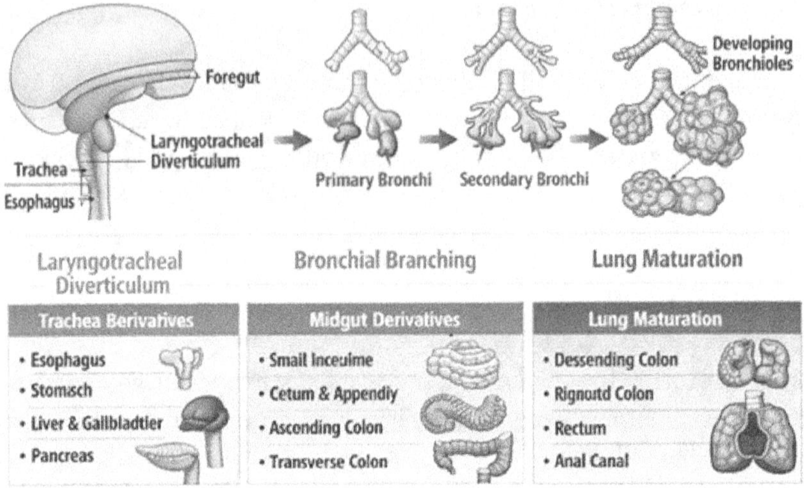

Development of the ***Respiratory System****, illustrating the sequential stages from the****laryngotracheal diverticulum to bronchial branching****and* ***lung maturation****. It shows:* ***Laryngotracheal Diverticulum:****the outpouching from the foregut forming thet rachea and esophagus.*
Bronchial Branching:*division into primary, secondary, and tertiary bronchi, establishing the lobar pattern.*
Lung Maturation:*progression through Pseudoglandular, canalicular, and alveolar stages, culminating in functional alveoli surrounded by capillaries.*

Histologic Stages of Lung Development

1. **Pseudoglandular Stage (Weeks 5–17)**: Branching resembles exocrine glands; terminal bronchioles form; no alveoli; gas exchange impossible.
2. **Canalicular Stage (Weeks 16–25)**: Respiratory bronchioles and alveolar ducts form; vascularization increases; Type II pneumocytes begin surfactant synthesis; limited gas exchange is possible late in this stage.
3. **Terminal Sac Stage (Week 24–Birth)**: Numerous terminal sacs form; capillaries closely appose alveolar epithelium; surfactant production increases; survival improves significantly.
4. **Alveolar Stage (Late Fetal Period–Childhood)**: Alveoli mature; most alveoli form postnatally, continuing until about eight years of age.

At birth, lungs contain amniotic fluid and secretions, cleared by thoracic compression, lymphatic absorption, and pulmonary circulation.

Surfactant and Neonatal Physiology

Surfactant, produced by Type II pneumocytes, lowers alveolar surface tension and prevents collapse. Production begins at weeks twenty to twenty-two, reaching adequate levels by thirty-four to thirty-six weeks. Corticosteroids accelerate pneumocyte maturation. Respiratory distress syndrome in premature infants results from insufficient surfactant, causing atelectasis and hypoxemia.

Congenital Anomalies

- **Esophageal Atresia with Tracheoesophageal Fistula**: Most common foregut anomaly; results from incomplete septation. Presents with polyhydramnios prenatally and choking, coughing, and cyanosis during feeds postnatally.
- **Isolated TEF or EA**: Rare variants causing recurrent aspiration or immediate regurgitation.
- **Pulmonary Hypoplasia**: Often secondary to congenital diaphragmatic hernia or oligohydramnios.
- **Laryngeal Atresia (CHAOS)**: Failure of recanalization, producing airway obstruction and enlarged echogenic lungs prenatally.

Chapter Summary

The respiratory system originates as a foregut diverticulum under RA, TBX4, and FGF10 signaling. Tracheoesophageal separation establishes the larynx, trachea, and esophagus. Bronchial branching and mesenchymal support form the bronchial tree. Lung maturation proceeds through the Pseudoglandular, canalicular, terminal sac, and alveolar stages. Surfactant production is critical for neonatal survival. EA/TEF and pulmonary hypoplasia exemplify congenital anomalies of respiratory development.

Self-Assessment Questions

1. Which germ layers give rise to the epithelium and the cartilage/smooth muscle of the tracheobronchial tree?
2. What molecular signals initiate lung development, and what abnormalities occur if they are disrupted?
3. Describe the stages of lung development and the viability of neonates born in each stage.
4. What is the embryologic basis of Esophageal atresia with distal tracheoesophageal fistula?
5. Why do infants with EA/TEF present with polyhydramnios prenatally and choking during feeds postpartum?
6. At what gestational age is surfactant production sufficient to support extrauterine life?

MCQs

1. The lung bud originates as an outgrowth from the:

A. Hindgut
B. Foregut
C. Midgut
D. Pharyngeal pouch

Answer: B

2. Failure of tracheoesophageal septation can lead to:

A. Pulmonary hypoplasia
B. Tracheoesophageal fistula
C. Congenital diaphragmatic hernia
D. Bronchiectasis

Answer: B

CHAPTER XV

Development of the Kidney and Ureter

Learning Objectives

By the end of this chapter, the student should be able to describe the embryologic origin of the urinary system from intermediate mesoderm, distinguish the pronephros, mesonephros, and metanephros and understand their developmental roles, explain how the ureteric bud and metanephric blastema interact to form the collecting system and nephron, describe kidney ascent, rotation, and changes in blood supply, recognize major congenital anomalies of the kidney and ureter, and understand the genetic basis of renal developmental disorders such as PAX2 and WT1 mutations.

Integrated Video Lecture

Video Title: Development of the Kidney and Ureter
Hyperlink: https://youtu.be/2ejdeEXZVmw
Source: Private institutional server

Origin of the Urinary System

The urinary system arises from intermediate mesoderm, which forms the urogenital ridge along the dorsal body wall. The nephrogenic cord, the lateral portion of this ridge, produces three successive renal systems in cranial-to-caudal sequence: pronephros, mesonephros, and metanephros. Only the metanephros persists as the permanent kidney.

Pronephros

Appearing in week four, the pronephros is the earliest and most cranial renal structure. It forms pronephric tubules and a pronephric duct but is nonfunctional and regresses by week five. Its role is purely as a developmental template.

Mesonephros

The mesonephros develops between weeks four and eight. It consists of mesonephric tubules and the mesonephric (Wolffian) duct. It functions briefly before regressing. In males, the mesonephric duct persists as the epididymis, ductus deferens, and ejaculatory duct. In females, it largely regresses, with remnants occasionally persisting as Gartner duct cysts. The mesonephros is essential for establishing the outflow tract that supports definitive kidney development.

Metanephros (Permanent Kidney)

The metanephros appears in week five and becomes the permanent kidney. It forms through reciprocal induction between the ureteric bud, an epithelial diverticulum from the caudal mesonephric duct, and the metanephric blastema, a mesodermal tissue cap. This interaction is critical for nephron formation.

Collecting System Development

The ureteric bud gives rise to the collecting system: ureter, renal pelvis, major and minor calyces, collecting ducts, and tubules. Branching morphogenesis proceeds in a stereotyped sequence, with early branches forming calyces and later branches forming ducts and tubules. The ureteric bud epithelium induces the blastema to form nephrons.

Nephron Development

Collecting tubules induce blastemal cells to form metanephric vesicles, which elongate into S-shaped tubules and differentiate into nephrons. Nephrons consist of Bowman's capsule, proximal tubule, loop of Henle, and distal tubule. Glomerular capillaries invade Bowman's capsule to form renal corpuscles. Nephron formation begins in week eight and continues until birth, but no new nephrons form postnatally.

Functional Maturation

By week ten, the metanephric kidney produces urine, contributing to amniotic fluid volume. The placenta continues to handle fetal waste, so fetal urine is not excretory but essential for fluid homeostasis.

Kidney Ascent and Rotation

Initially located in the pelvic region, the kidneys ascend to the lumbar region (T12–L2) due to differential growth. They rotate medially so the hilum faces inward. During ascent, kidneys acquire new blood supplies from progressively higher vessels, while lower vessels regress. Persistence of these vessels produces supernumerary renal arteries, which are clinically significant as end arteries.

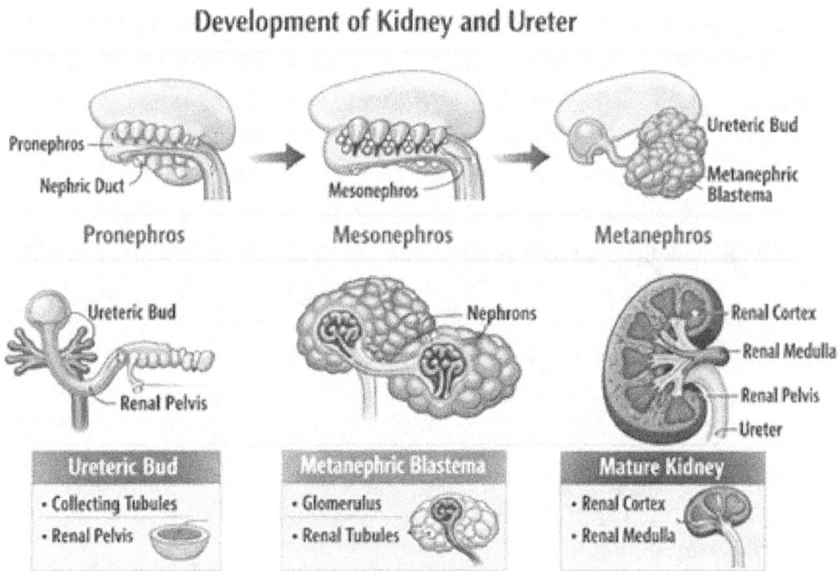

__Development of the Kidney and Ureter__, illustrating the sequential stages of __pronephros, mesonephros, and metanephros__ development. It shows how the __ureteric bud__ arises from the __mesonephric duct__, grows toward the __metanephric blastema__, and induces nephron formation. The lower panels highlight the __branching of the ureteric bud__ into collecting tubules, the differentiation of the __metanephric blastema__ into nephrons, and the structure of the __mature kidney__

with cortex, medulla, pelvis, and ureter continuity.

Congenital Anomalies

- **Renal Agenesis**: Unilateral agenesis is often asymptomatic; bilateral agenesis causes Potter sequence with oligohydramnios, limb deformities, flattened facies, and pulmonary hypoplasia.
- **Pelvic Kidney**: Failure of ascent leaves the kidney in the pelvis.
- **Horseshoe Kidney**: Fusion of lower poles traps the kidney under the inferior mesenteric artery; associated with Turner syndrome.
- **Rotational Anomalies**: Abnormal rotation alters hilum orientation.
- **Supernumerary Renal Arteries**: Persistence of transient vessels during ascent.
- **Polycystic Kidney Disease (PKD)**: Autosomal recessive PKD presents in infancy with collecting duct dilation; autosomal dominant PKD presents in adulthood.
- **Wilms Tumor**: A malignant childhood tumor arising from abnormal mesenchymal-epithelial transformation, often linked to WT1 mutations.
- **Renal Coloboma Syndrome**: PAX2 mutation causes renal hypoplasia and optic nerve abnormalities.

Development of the Ureter

The ureter arises from the ureteric bud. Its epithelium forms transitional urothelium, while smooth muscle and connective tissue derive from mesoderm. Proper bud formation and integration are essential for normal ureteral development.

Summary of Tissue Origins

Structure	Embryologic Origin
Collecting ducts, calyces, pelvis, ureter	Ureteric bud (intermediate mesoderm)
Nephrons (Bowman's capsule → distal tubule)	Metanephric blastema
Ureteric wall smooth muscle	Mesoderm of the ureteric bud
Transitional epithelium of the ureter/pelvis	Ureteric bud epithelium
Podocytes, tubular cells	Metanephric blastema

Chapter Summary

The urinary system develops from intermediate mesoderm through three sequential renal systems: pronephros, mesonephros, and metanephros. Permanent kidney development depends on reciprocal induction between the ureteric bud and metanephric blastema. The ureteric bud forms the collecting system, while the blastema forms nephrons. Kidneys ascend, rotate, and acquire new blood supplies. Congenital anomalies arise from disruptions in bud–blastema interactions, ascent, rotation, or genetic mutations such as PAX2 and WT1.

Self-Assessment Questions

1. What are the derivatives of the ureteric bud and the metanephric blastema?
2. Describe the embryologic basis of renal agenesis.
3. How does the blood supply to the kidneys change during ascent?
4. What is the significance of supernumerary renal arteries?
5. Explain the pathogenesis of Wilms' tumor in terms of embryologic cell populations.
6. Which gene defect leads to renal coloboma syndrome, and what organs are affected?

MCQs

1. The permanent kidney (metanephros) develops from:

A. Pronephros
B. Mesonephros
C. Metanephric blastema and ureteric bud
D. Cloaca

Answer: C

2. The paramesonephric (Müllerian) ducts give rise to:

A. Epididymis and vas deferens
B. Seminal vesicle and prostate
C. Uterus and fallopian tubes
D. Testis and scrotum

Answer: C

CHAPTER XVI

Development of the Urinary Bladder and Urethra

Learning Objectives

By the end of this chapter, the student should be able to describe the embryologic division of the cloaca into the anorectal canal and urogenital sinus, explain the origin and differentiation of the urinary bladder, describe the development of the male and female urethra including segmental origins, explain the formation and significance of the trigone of the bladder, and recognize the embryologic basis of urachal anomalies and bladder exstrophy.

Integrated Video Lecture

Video Title: Development of the Bladder and Urethra
Hyperlink: https://youtu.be/0leienKnvv8
Source: Private institutional server

The Cloaca and Urorectal Septum

At the caudal end of the embryo, the hindgut terminates in the cloaca, an endoderm-lined chamber in contact with the cloacal membrane. The cloaca receives the allantois ventrally and the hindgut dorsally. Between weeks four and seven, the Urorectal septum partitions the cloaca into a dorsal anorectal canal (rectum and upper anal canal) and a ventral urogenital sinus (urinary bladder, urethra, and genital ducts). Rupture of the cloacal membrane establishes the anus posteriorly and the urogenital opening anteriorly.

The Urogenital Sinus

The urogenital sinus differentiates into three regions:

- **Vesical part (cranial)** → urinary bladder
- **Pelvic part (middle)** → prostatic and membranous urethra in males; entire urethra in females

- **Phallic part (caudal)** → spongy urethra in males; vestibule of the vagina in females

Development of the Urinary Bladder

The bladder develops from the vesical part of the urogenital sinus. Endoderm forms the epithelial lining, while mesoderm contributes smooth muscle and connective tissue.

Trigone Formation: Incorporation of the caudal mesonephric ducts into the dorsal bladder wall creates the trigone. Although initially mesodermal, the trigone becomes endodermally lined.

Ureteral Separation: Initially, ureters open into the mesonephric ducts. As the bladder enlarges, the ureters acquire separate openings superior to the mesonephric ducts, explaining the adult arrangement of ureteral and ejaculatory duct orifices.

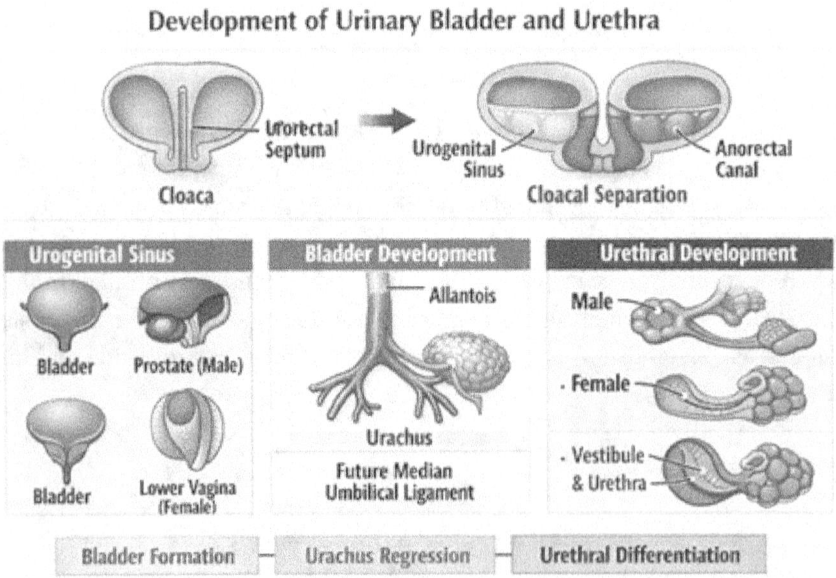

Development of the Urinary Bladder and Urethra, *illustrating the transformation of the* ***cloaca*** *into the* ***urogenital sinus*** *and* ***anorectal canal,*** *followed by the differentiation of the****bladder, urethra, and associated structures.*** *The diagram shows:*
Cloacal Separation: *division by the Urorectal septum into anterior (urogenital sinus) and posterior (anorectal canal) compartments.*
Bladder Development: *connection of the allantois to the developing bladder and regression of the urachus into the median umbilical ligament.*
Urethral Differentiation: *distinct pathways for male (penile urethra) and female (vestibule and urethra) development.*

The Allantois and Urachus

The bladder initially communicates with the allantois. This connection constricts to form the urachus, a fibrous cord linking the bladder apex to the umbilicus. In adults, the urachus becomes the median umbilical ligament.

Urachal Anomalies: Incomplete obliteration produces:

- Urachal fistula → patent tract with urine leakage at the umbilicus
- Urachal sinus → blind-ending remnant near the umbilicus
- Urachal cyst → cystic dilation along the tract

Development of the Urethra

Female Urethra: Entirely derived from endoderm of the urogenital sinus; surrounding tissues from mesoderm.

Male Urethra:

- **Prostatic urethra**: cranial portion from vesical part; caudal portion from pelvic part
- **Membranous urethra**: pelvic part of the sinus
- **Spongy urethra**: phallic part of the sinus, surrounded by corpus spongiosum
- **Distal urethra in glans**: ectodermal ingrowth from the glans tip canalizes and joins the endodermal urethra

Thus, most of the male urethra is endodermal, with the distal segment ectodermal.

Clinical Correlations

- **Bladder Exstrophy**: Failure of closure of the lower abdominal wall and anterior bladder wall exposes the posterior bladder mucosa. Often associated with epispadias.
- **Urachal Anomalies**: Persistent urachus produces fistulas, sinuses, or cysts.
- **Congenital Urethral Abnormalities**:
    - Hypospadias: ventral urethral opening due to failed urethral fold fusion
    - Epispadias: dorsal urethral opening, often with bladder exstrophy
    - Posterior urethral valves: obstructive membranes in the prostatic urethra, causing urinary obstruction in males

Chapter Summary

The urinary bladder and urethra develop from the urogenital sinus after cloacal division by the Urorectal septum. Bladder epithelium is endodermal, smooth muscle mesodermal. The trigone forms from incorporated mesonephric ducts. The urachus, a remnant of the allantois, may persist as cysts, sinuses, or fistulas. Urethral development is sex-specific: female urethra is entirely endodermal, while the male urethra has both endodermal and ectodermal origins. Bladder exstrophy and urachal anomalies exemplify congenital malformations linked to cloacal partitioning and abdominal wall closure.

Self-Assessment Questions

1. What structures arise from the three regions of the urogenital sinus?
2. How does the incorporation of the mesonephric ducts contribute to trigone formation?
3. What embryologic structure forms the median umbilical ligament in adults?

4. Describe the different embryologic origins of the male urethra.
5. What is the embryologic basis of bladder exstrophy?
6.
7. How do urachal cysts, sinuses, and fistulas differ anatomically?

MCQs

1. A newborn is noted to have urine leaking from the umbilicus. Imaging reveals a persistent tubular connection between the bladder and the umbilicus. Failure to obliterate which embryological structure is the most likely cause?

A. Vitelline duct
B. Urachus
C. Mesonephric duct
D. Paramesonephric duct
E. Allantoic diverticulum

Answer: B

Explanation:

The **urachus** is derived from the allantois and connects the fetal bladder to the umbilicus. Normally, it obliterates to form the **median umbilical ligament**. Persistence results in a **patent urachus**, leading to urine discharge from the umbilicus.

CHAPTER XVII

Development of the Male Reproductive System

Learning Objectives

By the end of this chapter, the student should be able to describe the origin of the testes from intermediate mesoderm and the gonadal ridge, explain the role of SRY, SOX9, testosterone, and Müllerian inhibiting substance (MIS/AMH) in male sexual differentiation, outline the development of the mesonephric duct and its derivatives, describe the process of testicular descent and the structures involved, explain the embryologic formation of the prostate, penis, scrotum, and male urethra, and recognize congenital anomalies including cryptorchidism, hypospadias, epispadias, persistent Müllerian duct syndrome, and androgen insensitivity syndrome.

Integrated Video Lecture

Video Title: Development of the Male Reproductive System
Hyperlink: https://youtu.be/fXxUaMaYxMY
Source: Private institutional server

Origins of the Male Reproductive System

The male reproductive system arises from intermediate mesoderm, forming the urogenital ridge. Three cell populations contribute to the testis: mesothelium (forming testis cords), underlying mesenchyme (forming connective tissue and Leydig cells), and primordial germ cells migrating from the yolk sac. Before week seven, the gonad is indifferent.

Genetic Switch for Male Development

The **SRY gene** on the Y chromosome encodes the testis-determining factor, which activates **SOX9**. SOX9 promotes Sertoli cell differentiation and induces AMH secretion, causing regression of Müllerian ducts. Leydig cells differentiate under hCG and pituitary influence, producing testosterone by week eight. Testosterone maintains mesonephric ducts, while conversion to dihydrotestosterone (DHT) drives external genitalia development.

Differentiation of the Testis

- **Testis cords**: arise from coelomic epithelium, containing germ cells and Sertoli cells; later form seminiferous tubules and rete testis.
- **Leydig cells**: interstitial mesenchyme producing testosterone.
- **Tunica albuginea**: fibrous capsule forming around the testis, more prominent than in the ovary.

Mesonephric Duct Derivatives

Testosterone stabilizes the mesonephric duct, forming efferent ductules, epididymis, ductus deferens, seminal vesicles, and ejaculatory ducts. Sertoli-derived AMH causes regression of Müllerian ducts. Vestigial remnants include the appendix, epididymis, and paradidymis.

Development of Male External Genitalia

By weeks four to five, mesenchymal proliferation forms the genital tubercle, urethral folds, and labioscrotal swellings. Under DHT influence:

- **Genital tubercle** elongates into the penis and glans.
- **Urethral folds** fuse ventrally to enclose the spongy urethra.
- **Labioscrotal swellings** fuse to form the scrotum, with the scrotal raphe marking the line of fusion.

Development of the Male Urethra

- **Endodermal origin**: prostatic, membranous, and spongy urethra (up to the glans) from the urogenital sinus.
- **Ectodermal origin**: distal glanular urethra from an ectodermal cord that canalizes and joins the endodermal urethra.

Thus, the urethra is predominantly endodermal, with an ectodermal terminal segment.

Development of the Prostate and Accessory Glands

- **Prostate**: endodermal buds from the prostatic urethra; mesenchyme forms stroma and smooth muscle.
- **Bulbourethral glands**: endodermal buds from the spongy urethra.
- **Seminal vesicles**: outgrowths of the mesonephric duct posterior to the bladder.

Testicular Descent

Testes descend in two phases:

1. **Abdominal descent**: guided by the gubernaculum, driven by differential growth.
2. **Inguinoscrotal descent**: influenced by testosterone, genitofemoral nerve signaling, and intra-abdominal pressure. The processus vaginalis precedes the testis into the scrotum, forming the tunica vaginalis. Failure of descent results in cryptorchidism.

Clinical Correlations

- **Hypospadias**: ventral urethral opening due to failed urethral fold fusion.
- **Epispadias**: dorsal urethral opening, associated with bladder exstrophy.
- **Cryptorchidism**: undescended testes, increasing risk of infertility and malignancy.
- **Persistent Müllerian Duct Syndrome**: MIS or receptor mutations cause persistence of female structures in XY males.
- **Androgen Insensitivity Syndrome**: androgen receptor mutation in XY individuals; external female phenotype, absent uterus, undescended testes.
- **Remnants**: appendix, epididymis, and paradidymis, clinically insignificant but exam-relevant.

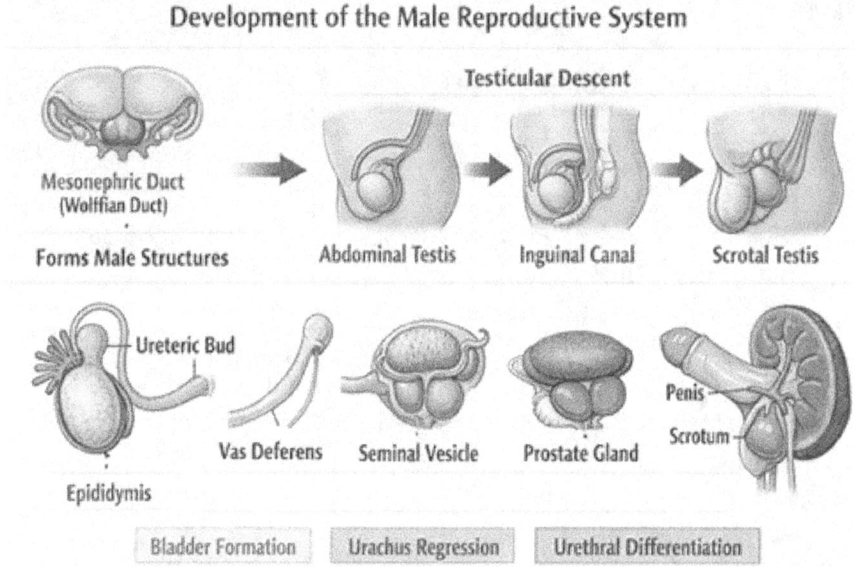

***Development of the Male Reproductive System**, illustrating the differentiation of the **mesonephric (Wolffian) duct** and the descent of the**testis.** The diagram shows:*

- ***Early Stage:** the undifferentiated gonad and mesonephric duct that give rise to male structures.*
- ***Testicular Descent:**guided by the**gubernaculum**, from the abdominal position through the inguinal canal into the scrotum.*
- ***Accessory Structures:** formation of the **epididymis, vas deferens, seminal vesicle, prostate gland,** and external genitalia **(penis and scrotum).***

Chapter Summary

Male differentiation requires SRY activation of SOX9, leading to Sertoli and Leydig cell pathways. Mesonephric duct derivatives form the epididymis, vas deferens, seminal vesicles, and ejaculatory ducts. DHT drives external genitalia formation. The urethra develops from both endoderm and ectoderm. Testes descend under gubernacular and hormonal guidance.

Congenital anomalies include hypospadias, epispadias, cryptorchidism, PMDS, and AIS.

Self-Assessment Questions

1. What are the roles of SRY, SOX9, MIS, and testosterone in male sexual differentiation?
2. Which structures derive from the mesonephric (Wolffian) duct?
3. Describe the formation of the male urethra and identify its endodermal and ectodermal components.
4. What is the embryologic basis of hypospadias and epispadias?
5. Explain the mechanism of persistent Müllerian duct syndrome.
6. Why do individuals with androgen insensitivity syndrome have female external genitalia but no uterus?

MCQs

1. A male infant is born with the urethral opening located on the ventral surface of the penis. This anomaly results from the failure of which developmental process?

A. Faulty fusion of the urethral folds
B. Formation of the genital tubercle
C. Development of labioscrotal swellings
D. Differentiation of mesonephric ducts
E. Regression of paramesonephric ducts

Answer: A

Explanation: This condition is **hypospadias**, caused by failure of the **urethral (urogenital) folds** to fuse, resulting in an abnormal ventral opening of the urethra.

2. A male infant is born with undescended testes. Which hormone is primarily responsible for the descent of the testes during development?

A. Follicle-stimulating hormone

B. Luteinizing hormone
C. Testosterone
D. Estrogen
E. Human chorionic gonadotropin

Answer: C

Explanation: **Testicular descent** is primarily mediated by **testosterone**, which influences the gubernaculum and guides the testes into the scrotum.

CHAPTER XVIII

Development of the Female Reproductive System

Learning Objectives

By the end of this chapter, the student should be able to describe the chronological development of the female reproductive system, explain the embryologic origin and differentiation of the ovaries, outline the development of the paramesonephric (Müllerian) ducts and their derivatives, describe the dual embryologic origin and innervation of the vagina, explain the development of the external genitalia, and correlate developmental errors with common congenital anomalies.

Integrated Video Lecture

Video Title: Development of the Female Reproductive System
Hyperlink: https://youtu.be/Cw7_w2FynfA
Source: Private institutional server

Introduction and Timeline of Sexual Differentiation

The female reproductive system develops from three embryologic components: the gonads, the paramesonephric ducts, and the primordium of the external genitalia. Genetic sex is determined at fertilization, but gonads remain morphologically indifferent until week six. Differentiation begins in week seven, with the external genitalia distinguishable by week twelve. Complete phenotypic differentiation is achieved by week twenty.

Genetic and Hormonal Basis of Female Differentiation

Initial gonadal development is identical in both sexes. In XX embryos, the absence of the Y chromosome and SRY gene means no testis-determining factor, testosterone, or Müllerian inhibiting substance. In this default pathway, the gonads differentiate into ovaries, Müllerian ducts persist, and female reproductive structures form.

Development of the Ovaries

Ovaries arise from coelomic epithelium, underlying mesenchyme, and primordial germ cells. Germ cells migrate from the yolk sac to the gonadal ridge. Primary sex cords degenerate, replaced by cortical cords that incorporate germ cells. These cords fragment into primordial follicles, each containing a primary oocyte surrounded by granulosa cells. Stromal cells derive from mesenchyme, and a tunica albuginea forms beneath the surface epithelium. Ovaries descend into the pelvis, guided by the gubernaculum, which later forms the ovarian and round ligaments.

Development of the Paramesonephric (Müllerian) Ducts

Paramesonephric ducts arise as invaginations of coelomic epithelium lateral to the urogenital ridge.

- Cranial unfused portions → uterine tubes
- Caudal fused portions → uterovaginal primordium → uterus, cervix, and upper third of the vagina

Development of the Vagina

The fused ducts contact the urogenital sinus, inducing sinovaginal bulbs. These form a solid vaginal plate that canalizes into the lower two-thirds of the vagina.

Dual Origin:

- Upper one-third → paramesonephric ducts
- Lower two-thirds → urogenital sinus

Innervation:

- Upper vagina → parasympathetic pelvic splanchnic nerves; sympathetic hypogastric plexus
- Lower vagina → pudendal nerve branches
  This explains differences in pain sensitivity between upper and lower segments.

Development of the External Genitalia

Mesenchymal proliferation around the urogenital membrane produces the genital tubercle, urethral folds, and labioscrotal swellings. In the absence of androgen:

- Genital tubercle → clitoris
- Urethral folds → labia minora
- Labioscrotal swellings → labia major

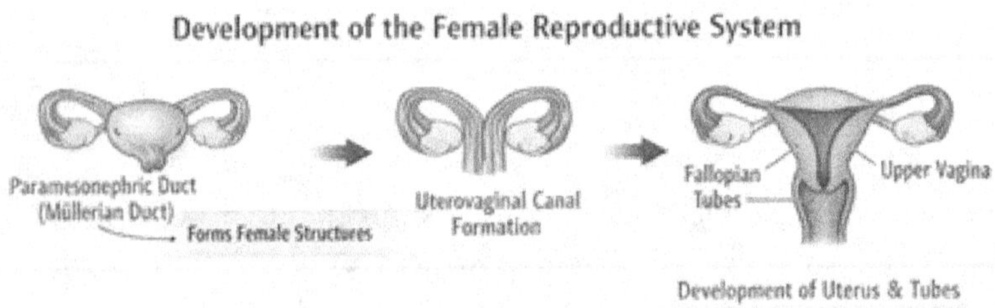

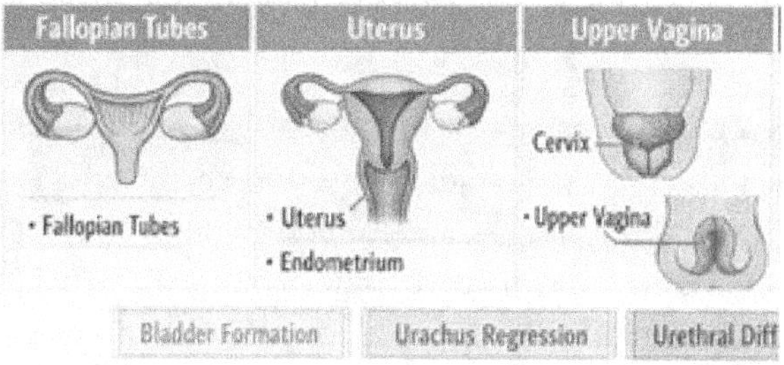

Development of the Female Reproductive System, illustrating the differentiation of the ***paramesonephric (Müllerian) ducts*** *into the* ***uterus, fallopian tubes, and upper vagina****. The diagram shows:*

- ***Early Stage:*** *the undifferentiated gonad and paired Müllerian ducts.*
- ***Uterovaginal Canal Formation:*** *fusion of the ducts in the midline.*
- ***Final Differentiation:*** *development of the* ***fallopian tubes, uterus, upper vagina****, and* ***external genitalia*** *(labia, clitoris, vulva).*

Congenital Anomalies and Clinical Correlations

- **Disorders of Sexual Development (Intersex)**: Often due to 21-hydroxylase deficiency, causing excess androgen and virilization of external genitalia, while internal organs remain female.
- **Müllerian Agenesis (MRKH Syndrome)**: Absence of uterus, cervix, and upper vagina; lower vagina present as a blind pouch.
- **Uterine Malformations**:
    - Unicornuate uterus: one duct develops
    - Bicornuate uterus: incomplete fusion
    - Uterus didelphys: complete failure of fusion, resulting in duplication
    - Septate uterus: failure of septum resorption after fusion

Chapter Summary

Female differentiation occurs in the absence of testis-determining signals. Ovaries develop from the gonadal ridge and germ cells. Paramesonephric ducts form the uterus, tubes, and upper vagina. The vagina has a dual embryologic origin and distinct innervation. External genitalia form without androgen influence. Errors in duct fusion or canalization produce characteristic anomalies such as a bicornuate or septate uterus.

Self-Assessment Questions

1. List the embryologic components involved in ovarian development.
2. Explain the dual origin of the vagina and its clinical relevance.
3. Identify the derivatives of the paramesonephric ducts.
4. Differentiate between a bicornuate uterus and a uterus didelphys.

MCQ / Vignette

1. A young woman presents with primary amenorrhea. Imaging reveals the absence of the uterus and upper vagina, but normal ovaries. Which embryological structure failed to develop?

A. Mesonephric duct
B. Paramesonephric duct
C. Genital tubercle
D. Urogenital sinus
E. Gonadal ridge

Answer: B

Explanation: This condition is consistent with **Müllerian agenesis (MRKH syndrome)**, due to failure of the **paramesonephric ducts**, which normally form the uterus, fallopian tubes, and upper vagina.

2. During development, failure of fusion of the paramesonephric ducts results in which anomaly?

A. Bicornuate uterus
B. Unicornuate uterus
C. Septate uterus
D. Vaginal atresia
E. Imperforate hymen

Answer: A

Explanation: Failure of **fusion of the paramesonephric ducts** leads to a **bicornuate uterus** (two uterine horns).

Part III – Craniofacial, Endocrine and Limb Development

CHAPTER XIX

Development of the Face and Palate

Learning Objectives

By the end of this chapter, the student should be able to describe the embryonic facial prominences and their contributions to definitive facial anatomy, explain the formation and fusion of the medial and lateral nasal prominences, outline the development of the primary and secondary palate, identify the mechanisms underlying cleft lip and cleft palate, and recognize major craniofacial anomalies resulting from failed fusion or migration of facial primordia.

Integrated Video Lecture
Video Title: Development of the Face and Palate
Hyperlink: https://youtu.be/ov2o_gL2Bjc
Source: Private institutional server

Origins of Facial Development

Between weeks four and eight, the face develops from neural crest–derived mesenchyme and pharyngeal arch mesoderm. Five facial prominences surround the primitive oral cavity (stomatodeum): the frontonasal prominence, paired maxillary prominences, and paired mandibular prominences. These swellings, covered by ectoderm, undergo coordinated growth and fusion to establish facial architecture.

Facial Prominences and Their Derivatives

- **Frontonasal prominence** → forehead, nasal bridge
- **Medial nasal prominences** → nasal septum, crest, tip of nose, philtrum, primary palate
- **Lateral nasal prominences** → alae of the nose
- **Maxillary prominences** → upper jaw, lateral upper lip, upper cheek
- **Mandibular prominences** → lower jaw, lower lip, lower cheek

Nasal placodes appear in week four, invaginate to form nasal pits, and generate medial and lateral nasal prominences.

Formation of the Lower Face

By week five, mandibular prominences fuse medially to form the mandible, lower lip, and lower face. Their dorsal portions contribute to maxillary prominences, establishing the first definitive facial boundary.

Fusion of Medial Nasal Prominences: Intermaxillary Segment

By week six, medial nasal prominences fuse to form the intermaxillary segment, which gives rise to the philtrum of the upper lip, four incisor teeth, and the primary palate (anterior to the incisive foramen).

Contribution of the Lateral Nasal Prominences

The lateral nasal prominences form the alae of the nose. Fusion with maxillary prominences traps ectodermal cells in the nasolacrimal groove, which canalize to form the nasolacrimal duct.

Growth and Final Shaping of the Face

From week eight onward, facial morphology refines through growth of the maxilla and mandible, descent of nasal pits, expansion of neural structures, and proportional elongation of the face relative to the neurocranium. Neural crest migration continues to shape midface and jaw structures.

Development of the Palate

Primary Palate (Weeks 4–7): Derived from the intermaxillary segment, forming the philtrum, premaxilla, and anterior palate.

Secondary Palate (Weeks 7–10): Palatine shelves from maxillary prominences initially grow vertically beside the tongue, then elevate horizontally as the mandible grows. They fuse along the midline to form the secondary palate and palatine raphe, joining anteriorly with the primary palate and superiorly with the nasal septum. This separates the oral and nasal cavities.

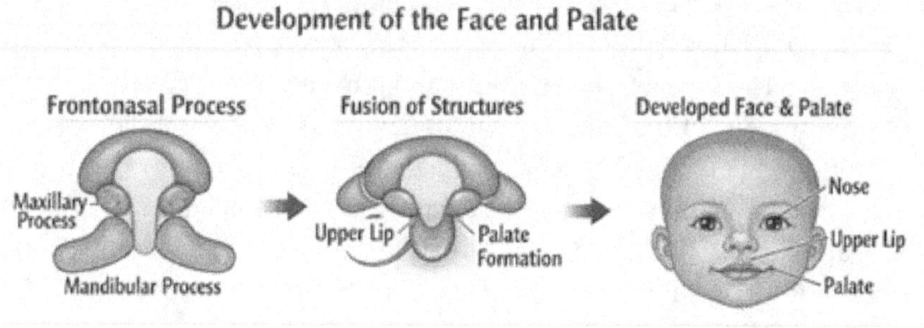

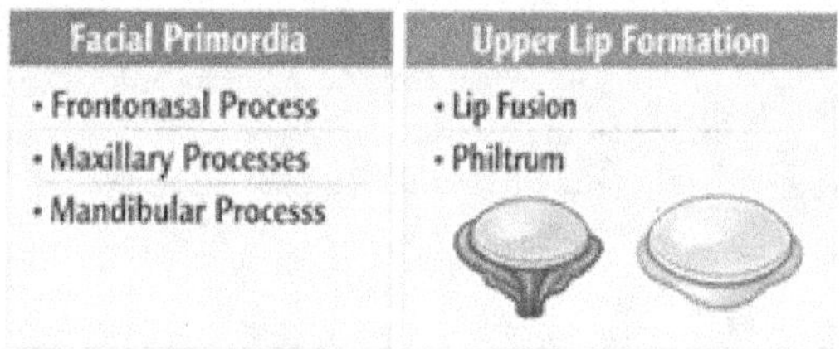

The Development of the Face and Palate, *illustrating the coordinated fusion of* ***the frontonasal, maxillary, and mandibular processes*** *to form the facial contours and palate.*
Facial Primordia: *the frontonasal process flanked by paired maxillary and mandibular processes.*
Fusion of Structures: *merging of these processes to form* ***the upper lip and primary palate,*** *with the philtrum marking the midline fusion.*
Palate Development: *differentiation into the* ***hard and soft palate,*** *completing the separation between the oral and nasal cavities.*

Clinical Correlations: Orofacial Clefts

- **Cleft Lip**: Failure of maxillary prominence to fuse with medial nasal prominence; may be unilateral, bilateral, or median.

- **Anterior Cleft Palate**: Failure of palatine shelves to fuse with the primary palate; often associated with cleft lip.
- **Posterior Cleft Palate**: Failure of palatine shelves to fuse with each other or the nasal septum; more common in females.
- **Combined Cleft Palate**: Involves both primary and secondary palates.
- **Oblique Facial Cleft**: Failure of fusion between lateral nasal, maxillary, and medial nasal prominences; exposes nasolacrimal duct.
- **Macrostomia (Lateral Facial Cleft)**: Incomplete fusion of maxillary and mandibular prominences, producing an abnormally wide mouth.

Mapping Facial Primordia to Adult Structures

Prominence	Adult Derivatives
Frontonasal	Forehead, nasal bridge
Medial nasal	Nasal septum, crest, tip, philtrum, primary palate
Lateral nasal	Alae of the nose
Maxillary	Upper jaw, lateral upper lip, upper cheek
Mandibular	Lower jaw, lower lip, lower cheek

Fusion lines between these regions correspond to sites of common clefts.

Chapter Summary

Facial development occurs through coordinated growth and fusion of five prominences derived from neural crest and pharyngeal arch mesoderm. Medial nasal prominences form the intermaxillary segment and primary palate, while palatine shelves from maxillary prominences create the secondary palate. Fusion events are critical for normal facial morphology. Cleft lip and palate arise from the failed fusion of specific prominences, and mapping embryonic origins helps predict congenital craniofacial anomalies.

Self-Assessment Questions

1. Which facial prominences contribute to the upper lip and philtrum?
2. How does the nasolacrimal duct form embryologically?
3. Differentiate between an anterior and posterior cleft palate.
4. What structures derive from the intermaxillary segment?

5. Explain the embryologic basis of macrostomia.

MCQs

1. The philtrum of the upper lip is formed by the fusion of:

A. Maxillary and mandibular processes
B. Frontonasal and maxillary processes
C. Mandibular and frontonasal processes
D. Lateral nasal and mandibular processes

Answer: B

2. Cleft palate results from failure of fusion of:

A. Maxillary and mandibular processes
B. Lateral nasal and maxillary processes
C. Palatine shelves
D. Frontonasal and mandibular processes

Answer: C

CHAPTER XX

Development of the Eye

Learning Objectives

By the end of this chapter, the student should be able to identify the germ layers contributing to ocular structures, explain the role of the optic vesicle and lens placode in early eye development, outline the formation of the optic cup and optic stalk, describe the differentiation of the retina, lens, and cornea, explain the development of the iris, ciliary body, sclera, and choroid, recognize congenital anomalies such as coloboma, anophthalmia, microphthalmia, and congenital cataract, and summarize key signaling pathways (Pax6, Shh, BMP, FGF) in ocular morphogenesis.

Integrated Video Lecture

Video Title: Development of the Eye
Hyperlink: https://youtu.be/2d5bVAp7hvM
Source: Private institutional server

Early Formation of the Eye (Week 4)

Eye development begins in the fourth week, when shallow optic grooves appear on the lateral walls of the forebrain. These grooves evaginate to form optic vesicles, hollow outpouchings of neuroectoderm. As the vesicles grow laterally, they contact the surface ectoderm, inducing it to thicken into the lens placode — the first step in lens formation.

Formation of the Optic Cup and Optic Stalk

Invagination of the optic vesicle produces the double-layered optic cup. The outer layer becomes the retinal pigment epithelium, while the inner layer differentiates into the neural retina. The optic stalk connects the optic cup to the forebrain and later transforms into the optic nerve. A ventral groove, the choroidal fissure, transmits the hyaloid artery and normally closes by the seventh week. Failure of closure results in coloboma, affecting the iris, retina, choroid, or optic nerve.

Tissue Contributions to Eye Development

- **Surface ectoderm:** lens, corneal epithelium, conjunctival epithelium.
- **Neuroectoderm:** neural retina, retinal pigment epithelium, epithelium of iris and ciliary body, sphincter and dilator pupillae, optic nerve fibers, glial cells.
- **Mesoderm:** choroid, sclera (with neural crest), extraocular muscles, connective tissue of ciliary processes.
- **Neural crest cells:** corneal stroma and endothelium, trabecular meshwork, scleral and choroidal components, iris stroma.

The anterior segment of the eye is largely derived from neural crest cells.

Development of the Retina

The optic cup's outer layer forms the retinal pigment epithelium, essential for photoreceptor function. The inner layer becomes the neural retina, differentiating into photoreceptors, bipolar cells, ganglion cells, and interneurons. Ganglion cell axons converge to form the optic nerve. The primitive intraretinal space between the two layers persists as a potential site for retinal detachment later in life.

Lens Development

The lens originates entirely from surface ectoderm under the influence of the optic vesicle. The lens placode invaginates to form a pit, then fuses to create the lens vesicle. Posterior cells elongate into primary lens fibers, while concentric secondary fibers establish the adult lens structure. Initially nourished by the hyaloid artery, the lens later depends on aqueous and vitreous humor after the artery regresses.

Development of the Optic Nerve

The optic stalk becomes the optic nerve as ganglion cell axons fill its lumen. The proximal hyaloid artery persists as the central artery of the retina. Failure of hyaloid regression leads to persistent fetal vasculature, impairing vision.

Development of the Iris and Ciliary Body

The iris develops from the anterior rim of the optic cup. Its epithelium and pupillary muscles derive from neuroectoderm, while the stroma originates from neural crest cells. The ciliary body arises from neuroectodermal epithelium, mesenchymal connective tissue, and ciliary processes, which produce aqueous humor and anchor the lens via zonule fibers.

Cornea, Choroid, and Sclera

The cornea forms from surface ectoderm (epithelium), mesoderm, and neural crest (stroma), and neural crest (endothelium). The choroid develops from mesenchyme, forming the vascular layer, while the sclera arises mainly from neural crest cells with mesodermal input.

Key Signaling Pathways in Ocular Morphogenesis

- Pax6: Master regulator of eye field specification; essential for lens induction and retinal differentiation.
- Shh: Provides midline signals, splitting the eye field into bilateral vesicles; mutations cause midline defects such as cyclopia.
- BMPs: Regulate ectodermal differentiation, lens induction, and corneal epithelium formation.
- FGFs: Promote lens placode invagination, retinal progenitor proliferation, and photoreceptor differentiation.

Disruption of these pathways can result in anomalies such as coloboma, microphthalmia, or congenital cataracts.

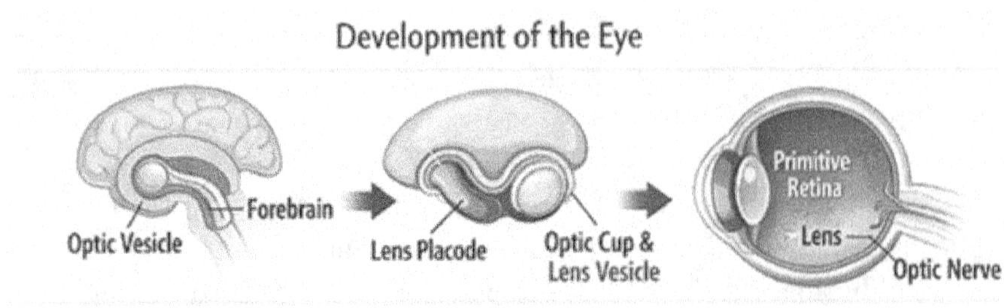

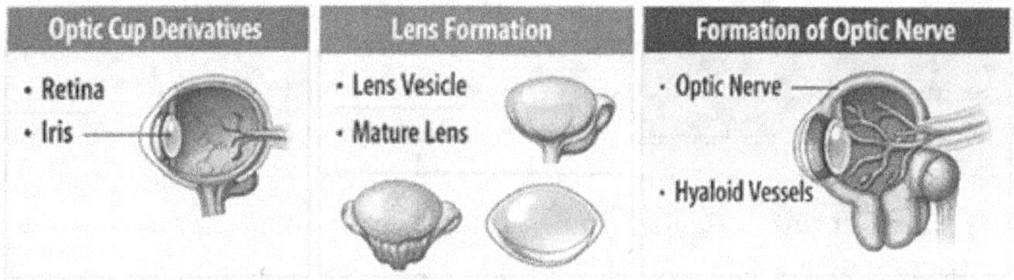

Development of the Eye, illustrating the sequential formation of the ***optic vesicle, lens placode****, and* ***optic cup****, leading to the mature eye structure. The diagram shows:*

Optic Vesicle Stage: *evagination from the forebrain contacting the surface ectoderm to form the lens placode.*

Optic Cup & Lens Vesicle: *invagination forming the double-layered optic cup (future retina) and the lens vesicle.*

Developing Eye: *differentiation into the* ***retina, lens, optic nerve****, and* ***hyaloid vessels.***

These coordinated events highlight the precision of inductive interactions, with disruptions leading to congenital anomalies such as coloboma or congenital cataract.

Clinical Correlations

- **Coloboma:** Incomplete closure of the choroidal fissure, producing keyhole-shaped iris defects; may extend to retina or optic nerve.
- **Congenital Retinal Detachment:** Failure of adhesion between neural retina and pigment epithelium.
- **Persistent Hyaloid Artery:** Leads to cataract, vitreous fibrosis, or retinal dysplasia.
- **Congenital Cataract:** Lens opacities due to infections (rubella), metabolic disorders (galactosemia), or genetic defects.
- **Aniridia:** Absence of iris from Pax6 mutations, often associated with poor foveal development.

Chapter Summary

Eye development begins with optic grooves that evaginate into optic vesicles, inducing lens formation and invaginating to form the optic cup. Surface ectoderm contributes the lens and corneal epithelium; neuroectoderm forms the retina, optic nerve, and iris epithelium; mesoderm forms vascular and fibrous layers; and neural crest cells contribute to cornea, sclera, choroid, and anterior segment structures. Closure of the choroidal fissure is essential to prevent coloboma. The intraretinal space predisposes to retinal detachment, while regression of the hyaloid artery is critical for normal lens and vitreous development.

Self-Assessment Questions

1. Which tissues contribute to the neural retina, RPE, and optic nerve?
2. Outline the steps in lens formation from the surface ectoderm.
3. What are the consequences of failed choroidal fissure closure?
4. Which embryonic layers contribute to corneal epithelium, stroma, and endothelium?
5. Describe the formation and later closure of the intraretinal space.
6. What abnormalities result from failure of hyaloid artery regression?

MCQs

1. The lens placode is induced by:

A. Optic vesicle
B. Neural crest cells
C. Surface ectoderm alone
D. Mesodermal condensation

Answer: A

2. Failure of optic fissure closure leads to:

A. Congenital cataract
B. Coloboma
C. Retinoblastoma
D. Microphthalmia

Answer: B

CHAPTER XXI

Development of the Tongue and Thyroid Gland

Learning Objectives

By the end of this chapter, the student should be able to identify the pharyngeal arch contributions to the anterior and posterior tongue, would be able describe the origin and migration of the thyroid diverticulum , would be able to explain the embryologic basis of C-cell formation and parathyroid embedding. The student would also recognize key landmarks such as the foramen cecum and terminal sulcus as also understand the origins of clinical anomalies such as thyroglossal duct cysts and ectopic thyroid tissue.

Integrated Video Lecture

Video Title: Development of the Tongue and Thyroid
Hyperlink: https://youtu.be/VRHOd_YrCjM
Source: Private institutional server

Development of the Tongue

The tongue begins to form in the floor of the primitive pharynx during the fourth week of development. Its mucosal components arise from pharyngeal arches, while its muscular elements originate from migrating occipital myotomes.

Anterior Two-Thirds (First Arch)

The oral tongue develops primarily from the first pharyngeal arch. The tuberculum impar appears as a median tongue bud, flanked by two lateral lingual swellings. These swellings enlarge rapidly, overgrow the tuberculum impar, and fuse at the midline to form the median sulcus. Together, they constitute the anterior two-thirds of the tongue.

Posterior One-Third (Third and Fourth Arches)

The posterior tongue is derived from the third and fourth arches. The second arch contributes to the copula, but this structure regresses. Overgrowth from arches three and four replaces it, with the third arch forming most of the posterior tongue and the fourth arch forming the epiglottic region.

Innervation Patterns

This embryologic origin explains the adult sensory innervation:

- Anterior two-thirds: general sensation via CN V3 (lingual nerve), taste via CN VII (chorda tympani).
- Posterior one-third: CN IX (glossopharyngeal).
- Epiglottic region: CN X (superior laryngeal branch).

Landmarks

The terminal sulcus marks the junction between the anterior and posterior tongue. At its apex lies the foramen cecum, the site of origin of the thyroglossal duct.

Muscular Development

Tongue muscles derive from occipital somite myoblasts that migrate into the developing tongue. These muscles are uniformly innervated by the hypoglossal nerve (CN XII), reflecting their somite-based origin.

Development of the Thyroid Gland

The thyroid is the first endocrine organ to develop, beginning in the fourth week.

Origin of the Thyroid Diverticulum

It arises as a midline endodermal diverticulum from the floor of the primitive pharynx, just caudal to the first arch, at the site of the future foramen cecum. This endodermal primordium gives rise to thyroid follicular cells.

Migration

The thyroid diverticulum descends ventral to the hyoid bone and laryngeal cartilages, maintaining a connection to the tongue via the thyroglossal duct. By the seventh week, the lobes reach their definitive position anterior to the second and third tracheal rings, joined by an isthmus. The thyroglossal duct normally degenerates, leaving only the foramen cecum as a remnant.

Cellular Contributions

- **Follicular cells:** endodermal origin; form thyroid follicles and secrete thyroid hormones (T3, T4).
- **Parafollicular (C) cells:** derived from neural crest cells via the ultimobranchial body (from the fifth pharyngeal pouch, often considered part of the fourth); secrete calcitonin.
- **Parathyroid glands:** superior parathyroids from the fourth pouch, inferior parathyroids from the third pouch; both embed on the dorsal thyroid surface.

Together, these structures establish the composite endocrine architecture of the neck.

Clinical Correlations

- **Thyroglossal Duct Cyst:** persistence of duct remnants along the migratory pathway; presents as a midline neck mass that moves with swallowing or tongue protrusion. Managed surgically with the Sistrunk procedure.
- **Ectopic Thyroid Tissue:** failure of normal migration may leave functional thyroid tissue at the tongue base (lingual thyroid) or other sites. In some cases, ectopic tissue is the only functioning thyroid.
- **Thyroid Agenesis or Hypoplasia:** abnormal primordium development causes congenital hypothyroidism (cretinism); early detection via neonatal screening is essential.
- **Aberrant Parathyroid Migration:** inferior parathyroids may descend excessively, sometimes into the mediastinum, complicating surgical management of hyperparathyroidism.

Chapter Summary

The tongue develops from multiple pharyngeal arches, with the anterior two-thirds derived from first-arch swellings and the posterior one-third from arches three and four. Its muscles originate from occipital somites and are innervated by CN XII. The thyroid begins as a midline diverticulum at the foramen cecum and migrates to its definitive location anterior to the trachea. Follicular cells are endodermal, while parafollicular cells arise from neural crest via the ultimobranchial body. Clinical anomalies such as thyroglossal duct cysts and ectopic thyroid tissue result from errors in migration or duct regression.

Self-Assessment Questions

1. Which pharyngeal arch derivatives form the anterior and posterior tongue?
2. What is the significance of the foramen cecum?
3. Describe the migration of the thyroid from its origin to its final position.
4. What are the embryologic origins of follicular cells and parafollicular (C) cells?
5. Why do thyroglossal duct cysts move with tongue protrusion?
6. How do the parathyroid glands reach the dorsal thyroid surface?

MCQs

1. Parafollicular (C-cells) of the thyroid are derived from:

A. Rathke's pouch
B. Ultimobranchial body
C. Neural crest cells
D. Thyroglossal duct

Answer: B

2. A 6-year-old child presents with a midline neck swelling that moves upward on protrusion of the tongue. The swelling is located just below the hyoid bone. This finding is most consistent with the persistence of which embryological structure

A. Pharyngeal pouch
B. Thyroglossal duct
C. Branchial cleft
D. Ultimobranchial body
E. Parathyroid primordium

Answer: B

Explanation: A **thyroglossal duct cyst** arises from the persistence of the thyroglossal duct, which normally degenerates after the thyroid gland descends from the foramen cecum to its final position.

CHAPTER XXII

Development of the Hypophysis Cerebri (pituitary gland)

Learning Objectives

By the end of this chapter, the student should be able to describe the dual embryologic origin of the pituitary gland ,explain the formation of Rathke's pouch and its derivatives , outline the development of the neurohypophysis from the diencephalon, identify the major components of adenohypophysis and neurohypophysis and also recognize congenital anomalies arising from abnormal pituitary development.

Integrated Video Lecture
Video Title: Development of the Hypophysis Cerebri
Hyperlink: https://youtu.be/tQVeSYqgmxU
Source: Private institutional server

Section 1 — Overview of Pituitary Development

The pituitary gland (hypophysis cerebri) develops from two distinct embryologic sources:

1. Oral ectoderm from the roof of the primitive mouth → Adenohypophysis (anterior pituitary)
2. Neuroectoderm from the floor of the diencephalon → Neurohypophysis (posterior pituitary)

Although these components become closely apposed, their embryologic origins, architecture, and functions remain distinct throughout life.

Section 2 — Formation of Rathke's Pouch (Anterior Pituitary)

Origin

Near the buccopharyngeal membrane, the roof of the primitive mouth (stomodeum) forms a finger-like ectodermal diverticulum:

- This diverticulum grows dorsally toward the developing brain.
- It is known as Rathke's pouch.

Growth and Differentiation

As Rathke's pouch elongates:

- Its connection to the oral cavity degenerates.
- Its anterior wall proliferates to form the pars distalis (the major endocrine portion).
- Its posterior wall contributes to the pars intermedia.
- Extensions around the infundibular stalk form the pars tuberalis.

Final Derivatives of Rathke's Pouch

Component	Description
Pars distalis	Largest anterior lobe; contains hormone-secreting cells (GH, ACTH, TSH, LH, FSH, PRL).
Pars tuberalis	Sleeve-like structure surrounding the infundibulum.
Pars intermedia	Thin epithelial zone; often separated from the pars distalis by a persistent cleft (hypophyseal cleft).

Section 3 — Development of the Neurohypophysis (Posterior Pituitary)

Simultaneously, the neuroectoderm of the diencephalon forms a ventral downward extension:

- This evagination becomes the infundibulum, comprising:
    - Infundibular stalk (pituitary stalk)
    - Pars nervosa (terminal expansion)

Functional Neurohypophysial Components

Component	Origin	Function
Pars nervosa	Neuroectoderm	Stores and releases **oxytocin** and **ADH** (synthesized in hypothalamus).
Infundibular stalk	Neuroectoderm	Connects pars nervosa to the hypothalamus; pathway for hypothalamic axons.
Median eminence	Superior part of neurohypophysis	Contains releasing/inhibiting hormones entering the hypophyseal portal system.

The hypothalamic nuclei (paraventricular and supraoptic) send axons through the stalk into the pars nervosa.

Section 4 — Integration of Anterior and Posterior Pituitary

As development progresses:

- Rathke's pouch and the infundibulum grow into close apposition.
- Despite this close relationship, the anterior and posterior lobes retain separate blood supplies and functional roles.
- The hypophyseal portal system develops from vascular channels of the median eminence and pars tuberalis, allowing hypothalamic regulation of the anterior pituitary.

Section 5 — Clinical Correlations

Rathke's Cleft Cyst

- Arises from persistent remnants of the cleft between the pars distalis and pars intermedia.
- Benign cystic lesion; may cause headache, visual disturbances, or pituitary dysfunction due to compression.

Craniopharyngioma

A clinically significant tumor thought to arise from epithelial remnants of Rathke's pouch.

Characteristics:

- Often calcified
- Frequently occurs in children or adolescents
- May cause visual field defects (compression of optic chiasm)
- Causes endocrine dysfunction by disrupting the pituitary or hypothalamus

Pituitary Agenesis or Hypoplasia

- Failure of the development of Rathke's pouch or infundibulum
- Results in congenital hypopituitarism
- May present with growth failure, adrenal insufficiency, or neonatal hypoglycemia

Ectopic Posterior Pituitary

- Neurohypophysis fails to migrate completely
- Appears as "bright spot" on MRI located outside the Sella turcica
- Often associated with pituitary stalk interruption syndrome

Chapter Summary

- The pituitary gland develops from two embryologic structures:

- **Rathke's pouch** (oral ectoderm) → anterior pituitary
- **Infundibular evagination** (neuroectoderm) → posterior pituitary

- Pars distalis, pars intermedia, and pars tuberalis arise from Rathke's pouch.
- Pars nervosa, median eminence, and infundibular stalk arise from neuroectoderm.
- The hypophyseal portal system enables hypothalamic control of anterior pituitary hormone secretion.
- Developmental anomalies include Rathke's cleft cysts, craniopharyngiomas, pituitary agenesis, and ectopic posterior pituitary.

Self-Assessment Questions

1. What are the two embryologic origins of the pituitary gland?
2. Which structures derive from Rathke's pouch?
3. What are the components of the neurohypophysis, and what is their function?
4. How does the hypophyseal portal system support anterior pituitary function?
5. What is the embryologic basis of craniopharyngioma?
6. How does a Rathke's cleft cyst differ from an ectopic posterior pituitary?

MCQs

1. The adenohypophysis develops from:

A. Rathke's pouch
B. Neurohypophysial bud
C. Ultimobranchial body
D. Foramen cecum

Answer: A

2. A tumor is found in the anterior pituitary of a young adult. Histological examination reveals origin from oral ectoderm. Which embryological structure gave rise to this part of the gland?

A. Infundibulum
B. Rathke pouch
C. Neural crest
D. Diencephalon
E. Primitive streak

Answer: B

Explanation:

The **anterior pituitary** develops from **Rathke's pouch**, an ectodermal outpocketing from the roof of the primitive oral cavity (stomodeum).

CHAPTER XXIII

Development of the Limbs

Learning Objectives

By the end of this chapter, the student should be able to:

- Describe the timeline of upper and lower limb formation.
- Identify the contributions of lateral plate mesoderm, somites, and neural crest cells.
- Explain the roles of the apical ectodermal ridge (AER), zone of polarizing activity (ZPA), HOX genes, and FGF signaling in limb patterning.
- Understand the mechanisms of limb rotation and their adult anatomical consequences.
- Recognize major congenital limb anomalies and their embryologic basis.

Integrated Video Lecture
Video Title: Development of Limbs
Hyperlink: https://youtu.be/8N0KWGoFVLY
Source: Private institutional server

Early Limb Development (Weeks 4–8)

Limb development begins toward the end of the fourth week, when paddle-shaped buds emerge from the lateral body wall. The upper limb buds appear first, around days 26–27, opposite the lower cervical and upper thoracic somites (C5–T1). The lower limb buds follow approximately two days later, opposite the lumbar and upper sacral somites (L1–S2). By the sixth week, a cartilaginous model is established, and between weeks 9–12, primary ossification centers become visible. Externally, limb development is essentially complete by the eighth week.

Tissue Origins of the Limb

Each limb bud contains a mesenchymal core derived from the lateral plate mesoderm, surrounded by surface ectoderm. The mesenchyme gives rise to bones, cartilage, tendons, blood vessels, and connective tissue, while the ectoderm covers the bud and forms specialized signaling structures such as the apical ectodermal ridge. Somites contribute myoblasts that form limb musculature and dermal cells that establish the dermis. Neural crest cells provide sensory nerves, Schwann cells, melanocytes, and connective tissue elements.

Limb Patterning Axes and Signaling Centers

Limb formation is organized along three axes: proximal–distal, anterior–posterior, and dorsal–ventral. Two signaling centers orchestrate this process.

- **Apical Ectodermal Ridge (AER):** Located at the distal tip of the limb bud, the AER secretes fibroblast growth factors (FGF2, FGF4, FGF8), stimulating mesenchymal proliferation and maintaining the progress zone for continuous outgrowth. Loss of the AER at any stage leads to truncation of limb elements.
- **Zone of Polarizing Activity (ZPA):** Found at the posterior margin of the limb bud, the ZPA secretes Sonic hedgehog (SHH), establishing the anterior–posterior axis. Disturbances in ZPA signaling can result in polydactyly or mirror-image duplication.
- **HOX Genes:** These gene clusters specify limb position and segment identity (stylopod, zeugopod, autopod). Disruption may cause loss or duplication of specific segments.

Formation of Bones, Joints, and Muscles

By the sixth week, mesenchyme differentiates into hyaline cartilage models, which are later replaced by bone through endochondral ossification. Primary ossification centers appear between weeks 9 and 12, and radiologists use ossification timing to estimate bone age. Joints form around day 51, when mesenchymal condensations cavitate to create synovial joints. Limb muscles arise from somite-derived myoblasts, with motor axons entering early and sensory fibers following.

Formation of Hand and Foot Plates

Around day 33, the distal limb flattens into hand plates, later mirrored by foot plates. Digital rays appear in the sixth week as mesenchymal condensations. Apoptosis between these rays separates the digits; failure of this process results in syndactyly. Limb segmentation follows a definitive sequence: stylopod (humerus/femur), zeugopod (radius–ulna/ tibia–fibula), and autopod (hand/foot).

Rotation of the Limbs (Week 7)

During the seventh week, the upper and lower limbs undergo opposite rotations. The upper limb rotates 90° laterally, positioning the elbows posteriorly and the extensor compartment dorsally. The lower limb rotates 90° medially, orienting the knees anteriorly and the extensor compartment ventrally. These rotations explain the adult dermatomal spiraling and compartmental arrangement of muscles and nerves.

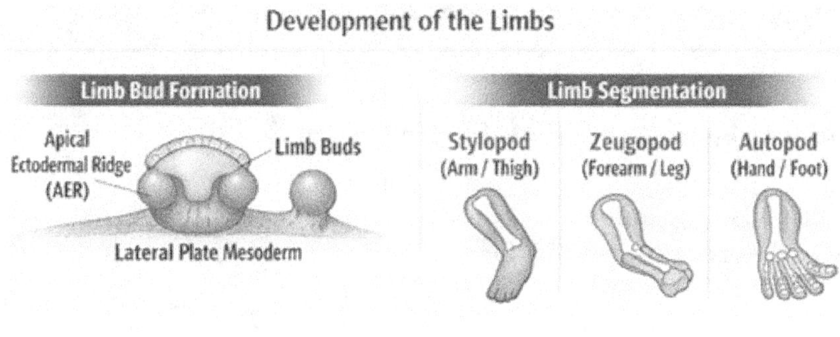

Development of the Limbs*, illustrating the sequential formation and differentiation of the* ***upper and lower limb buds****.*
Limb Bud Formation: *emergence from the lateral plate mesoderm with ectodermal covering and the* ***apical ectodermal ridge (AER)*** *guiding outgrowth.*
Segmentation: *differentiation into* ***stylopod (arm/thigh)****,* ***zeugopod***

***(forearm/leg)**, and **autopod (hand/foot)** regions.*
***Rotation:** opposite rotations of limbs — upper limb rotates **laterally**, lower limb **medially**, aligning flexor and extensor surfaces appropriately.*
***Final Patterning:** formation of digits through **apoptosis in interdigital zones**, establishing the definitive limb structure.*

Clinical Correlations: Limb Anomalies

Congenital limb anomalies occur in approximately 1 in 200 live births. They may result from genetic disruptions, teratogens such as thalidomide, or vascular insults.

- **Amelia / Meromelia:** Complete or partial absence of a limb, often due to early AER loss or vascular disruption.
- **Phocomelia:** Severe shortening with hands or feet attached close to the trunk, classically seen in thalidomide embryopathy.
- **Polydactyly:** Extra digits caused by abnormal SHH/ZPA signaling.
- **Syndactyly:** Failure of apoptosis between digital rays, leading to cutaneous or osseous fusion.
- **Clubfoot (Talipes Equinovarus):** A multifactorial condition characterized by adduction, inversion, and plantar flexion of the foot, often due to abnormal positioning or neuromuscular imbalance rather than primary developmental failure.

Chapter Summary

Limb buds arise in the fourth week from lateral plate mesoderm, covered by ectoderm, with contributions from somites and neural crest cells. The AER regulates proximal–distal outgrowth, the ZPA establishes anterior–posterior patterning, and HOX genes specify segment identity. Limb rotation during the seventh week produces adult anatomical orientation. Digital rays form through mesenchymal condensation and apoptosis, establishing fingers and toes. Congenital anomalies arise from disruptions in signaling centers, apoptosis, or vascular integrity.

Self-Assessment Questions

1. What are the three major axes of limb patterning, and which signaling centers regulate them?
2. Which tissues contribute to bones, muscles, dermis, and nerves of the limb?
3. How does the AER regulate limb outgrowth, and what happens if it is disrupted?
4. What embryologic events explain the opposite rotation of the upper and lower limbs?
5. Distinguish between phocomelia, meromelia, and amelia.
6. What is the embryologic basis of syndactyly and polydactyly?

MCQs

1. The apical ectodermal ridge (AER) is essential for:

A. Neural tube closure
B. Limb outgrowth and patterning
C. Somite segmentation
D. Placental formation

Answer: B

2. Digits are formed by:

A. Mesenchymal condensation
B. Apoptosis in interdigital zones
C. Rotation of limb buds
D. Fusion of limb ridges

Answer: B

CHAPTER XXIV

Birth Defects (Congenital Anomalies)

Learning Objectives

By the end of this chapter, the student should be able to define congenital anomalies and classify their causes, distinguish between genetic, chromosomal, and environmental factors, explain multifactorial inheritance in congenital disorders, identify major teratogens and their mechanisms, and correlate embryologic timing with clinical outcomes.

Integrated Video Lecture

Video Title: Birth Defects: Genetic and Environmental Basis
Hyperlink: https://youtu.be/6YxXl1yBi9U
Source: Private institutional server

Introduction

Congenital anomalies, or birth defects, are structural or functional abnormalities present at birth. They result from complex interactions between genetic predisposition and environmental influences during critical developmental periods. These anomalies are a leading cause of infant morbidity, mortality, and long-term disability worldwide.

Genetic Factors

Single-Gene Mutations

- Follow Mendelian inheritance patterns.
- Examples: cystic fibrosis, sickle cell anemia, Duchenne muscular dystrophy.
- Recurrence risks are predictable within families.

Polygenic Inheritance

- Traits influenced by multiple genes.
- Examples: cleft lip and palate, neural tube defects.
- Do not follow simple Mendelian ratios; expression is variable.

Multifactorial Inheritance

- Genetic susceptibility combined with environmental triggers.
- Accounts for 20–25% of congenital anomalies.
- Examples: congenital heart defects, clubfoot, some neural tube defects.

Chromosomal Aberrations

Numerical Abnormalities (Aneuploidy)

- Result from meiotic nondisjunction.
- Examples: trisomy 21 (Down syndrome), trisomy 18 (Edwards syndrome), monosomy X (Turner syndrome).
- Major contributors to spontaneous abortions.

Structural Abnormalities

- Include deletions, duplications, translocations, and inversions.
- Example: 22q11.2 deletion syndrome (DiGeorge syndrome).
- Chromosomal abnormalities account for ~15% of birth defects.

Teratogens (Environmental Factors)

Chemical Agents

- Alcohol → fetal alcohol spectrum disorders
- Thalidomide → limb reduction defects

- Anticonvulsants, isotretinoin → craniofacial and neural anomalies

Infectious Agents

- TORCH infections (Toxo
- plasma, Rubella, CMV, HSV)
- Zika virus → microcephaly

Physical Agents

- Ionizing radiation → growth retardation, microcephaly
- Hyperthermia → neural tube defects

Environmental teratogens account for ~10% of congenital anomalies, often amplified in genetically susceptible individuals.

Clinical Integration: High-Yield Concepts

- Teratogenic effects depend on **dose, timing, and genotype**.
- The **embryonic period (weeks 3–8)** is most vulnerable, as organogenesis occurs.
- Multifactorial disorders show population-specific recurrence risks, emphasizing the importance of genetic counseling.

Chapter Summary

Congenital anomalies arise from genetic, chromosomal, environmental, or combined causes. Multifactorial inheritance is common and clinically significant. Chromosomal abnormalities are a major cause of pregnancy loss. Prevention strategies include genetic counseling, prenatal screening, and avoidance of known teratogens during critical developmental windows.

Key Learning Points

- Aneuploidy commonly results from meiotic nondisjunction.
- Polygenic traits do not follow Mendelian inheritance.
- Environmental effects are strongest during weeks 3–8 of embryogenesis.

Self-Assessment Questions

1. Define congenital anomalies and classify their causes.
2. Differentiate between single-gene, polygenic, and multifactorial inheritance.
3. What are the most common chromosomal abnormalities associated with birth defects?
4. List major teratogens and describe their mechanisms of action.
5. Why is the embryonic period (weeks 3–8) considered the most vulnerable to teratogens?

About This E-book

Clinical Embryology is a Video-Integrated Learning Resource that offers a modern and accessible approach to mastering the science of human development. Structured across twenty-four chapters and enriched with integrated video lectures, the book guides students from the earliest stages of gametogenesis through the complexities of congenital anomalies. Each section is carefully designed to simplify intricate concepts, connect them to clinical practice, and reinforce understanding through clear explanations and self-assessment opportunities. This resource is particularly valuable for undergraduate medical students preparing for examinations such as the USMLE and NBME, yet its scope extends to learners worldwide who seek clarity in developmental biology.

By combining foundational principles with clinical relevance, it transforms embryology from an abstract subject into a practical and engaging journey. With its blend of scholarly rigor and student-friendly narration, the book empowers aspiring physicians to approach embryology with confidence, curiosity, and a deeper appreciation of its role in medicine

About The Author

Dr. Shrikant Akolekar is an academic author and educator with extensive experience in teaching undergraduate medical students. He has devoted his career to bridging foundational science with clinical practice, guiding learners through genetics, developmental biology, and neuroanatomy with precision and clarity.

As the creator and narrator of this video-integrated textbook, Dr. Akolekar blends scholarly rigor with student-friendly explanations, reflecting his commitment to accessible, high-quality medical education. His work continues to inspire aspiring physicians to approach embryology not merely as an academic requirement, but as a vital key to understanding human health and disease.

www.ingramcontent.com/pod-product-compliance
Lightning Source LLC
LaVergne TN
LVHW022222200926
848481LV00006B/2069
* 9 7 9 8 9 0 4 7 9 9 9 5 3 *